mHealth

Global Opportunities and Challenges

Colin Konschak, MBA, FHIMSS
Dave Levin, M.D.
William H. Morris, M.D.

FOREWORD BY
Geeta Nayyar, M.D., MBA

This publication is intended to provide accurate and authoritative information in regard to the subject matter covered. The statements and opinions expressed in this book are those of the authors.

ISBN-13: 978-0-9834824-1-3
ISBN-10: 0983482411

Convurgent Publishing, LLC
4445 Corporation Lane, Suite #227
Virginia Beach, VA 23462
Phone: (877) 254-9794, Fax: (757) 213-6801
Website: www.convurgent.com   Email: info@convurgent.com

Special Orders.

Bulk Quantity Sales. Special discounts are available on quantity purchases of 25 or more copies by corporations, government agencies, academic institutions, and other organizations. Please contact Convurgent Publishing's Sales Department at sales@convurgent.com or at the address above.

Library of Congress Control Number: 2013915633
Bibliographic data:

mHealth Opportunities and Challenges / Colin Konschak, Dave Levin, William H. Morris
p. cm.

1. mHealth strategy. 2. Electronic health records. 3. Mobile health. 4. Health information technology. 5. Global eHealth. 6. Patient engagement. 7. Accountable care organizations. 8. Personal health records.

ISBN: 978-0-9834824-1-3

Credits
Cover Design: Keri DeSalvo
Copyediting: J.M. Bohn, Marcia Cronin

ABOUT THE AUTHORS

Colin Konschak, MBA, FACHE, FHIMSS, is the managing partner and CEO of the Virginia Beach, Va.-based management consulting firm, Divurgent.

Dave Levin, M.D., is chief medical information officer at Cleveland Clinic. He has more than 25 years experience in medical operations, information systems, and strategic planning for healthcare transformation.

William H. Morris, M.D., is associate chief medical information officer at the Cleveland Clinic and a practicing hospitalist in the clinic's Medicine Institute.

ACKNOWLEDGMENTS

Dave Levin, M.D.

I would like to start by thanking my fellow authors, Will Morris and Colin Konschak, and our corresponding author, Debra Gordon. When we decided the four of us would work together on this book, we weren't sure if the experience would be insanely great or just insane. In retrospect it was probably both. I can honestly say it was a pleasure and honor to work with such creative and dedicated partners.

Thanks also to my wife, Beth Ezzell Levin, M.D., my partner in all things personal and professional. If not for her support and advice, I would not be where I am today, and this book would just be a dream. Thanks for following me down Mount Tremont and into our lives together.

Finally, I would like to thank my mentors and colleagues, especially those at the Cleveland Clinic and those who generously contributed to this book. You have been an important part of my professional life and helped me in countless ways over the years. The field of medical informatics is still in its infancy—an "undiscovered country" of sorts. Thank you to all who have shed some light on the path forward.

William H. Morris, M.D.

First, I would like to thank my loving wife, Keira, and my children, Holden, Haley, and Lexi, for their support, guidance, inspiration, and humor.

I am deeply grateful to the Cleveland Clinic for providing me with the opportunity to practice medicine among such inspiring caregivers. Working together with them to provide the best possible patient care is a blessing.

Thanks to my Clinical Informatics colleagues, who perpetually push for tools that will best serve patient care. I am especially grateful to Brent Hicks, Beth Meese, Mat Coolidge, Dale Pickle, and the rest of the CSC and CSO team. I thank you and honor you.

Finally, I wholeheartedly thank my fellow authors, Colin and Dave, and writer, Debra. Count me in for round two.

Colin Konschak, MBA, FACHE, FHIMSS

I would like to thank various people and organizations for their contributions to this text. Without their involvement, this project would have never gotten off the ground. Thanks to my employer, Divurgent, for providing a very generous grant to seed this project, along with the space to bring it to fruition. Thanks also to Debra Gordon, our corresponding author, who was able to take our thoughts and writing and turn it into something quite outstanding. Thanks to Keri DeSalvo for her help with graphic design, including our cover.

Thanks to Dr. Geeta Nayyar for writing the foreword and introducing us to numerous industry experts, and, of course, thanks to those experts for their thoughts, quotes, research, etc., which can be found throughout the book. Many thanks to J.M. Bohn, for everything done to finalize our content and bring this project across the finish line. Lastly, thanks to Convurgent Publishing for giving us this opportunity and all that it did to bring our book to market.

Table of Contents

Foreword. mHealth: It's Personal

Mobile technology touches every aspect of our daily lives as a society, from the minute our day starts—often with the alarm clocks on our phones waking us—to managing our day using our mobile calendars. We have come to rely on our mobile devices, whether to communicate with colleagues or loved ones through emails, texts, or social media, or to access information at our fingertips, whether online or through applications, files, photos, or videos stored on our devices. There is no doubt that mobile technology has made the world a smaller and easier place to navigate.

Enter the mobile phone into health care. It seems natural that this smart technology would be an important linkage in the healthcare environment, which is fraught with disconnected systems and stakeholders.

Today's mobile technology touches every aspect of the global healthcare system. Patients can make appointments, check their medical records, and receive care reminders on their mobile phones. Physicians use tablets and laptops to access electronic medical records (EMRs), review diagnostic scans, and write e-prescriptions. Hospitals and healthcare systems are expanding their service "footprints" through telemedicine and telehealth initiatives.

These are just a few of the ways mobile devices, applications, and networks are changing the nation's healthcare system, raising new challenges while opening the door to new opportunities for all types of participants. New advances in mobile technology are announced daily, and the pace of change is accelerating. Clearly, we are in the early stages of the mHealth revolution—a dramatic transformation of the global healthcare landscape.

This publication, *mHealth: Global Opportunities and Challenges*, provides a practical guide for patients, providers, payers, and other healthcare enterprises making plans for the future. It covers the key aspects of mHealth, including:

- Mobile devices, such as smart phones, tablets, laptops, kiosks, interactive robots, and medical carts;

- Mobile applications for patients, physicians, hospitals, and other participants;

- Smart sensors for monitoring prosthetic implants and devices;

- Wireless networks that provide real-time access to clinical and business data from virtually any location;

- Telehealth and telemedicine programs that remove geographic restrictions on service delivery;

- "Big data" collection and analysis programs for improved business intelligence, simulations, and predictive modeling; and

- Emerging opportunities for healthcare technology companies and service providers.

Individually, these mHealth devices, applications, and systems enhance the communication capabilities of patients, providers, payers, and other participants. Collectively, they break down the walls of the traditional in-person healthcare delivery system. While patients will still need to see providers for many types of diagnostic, treatment, and follow-up services, more and more encounters will occur in a mobile setting—at home, in the workplace, in the car, or while traveling.

Taking advantage of the mHealth trend will require many enterprises to invest in their networks and other infrastructure systems. They will need to analyze, pilot, and deploy new mobile devices and applications and strengthen their public and provider communications and marketing programs. Most importantly, mHealth will require enterprises to adopt new ways of thinking about virtually every aspect of healthcare services, from the first patient contact to the final billing and collection.

These mHealth systems and technologies may provide the key to delivering truly personalized clinical care, while supporting individual wellness and disease-prevention programs. In addition, mHealth initiatives can accelerate operational and business processes and reduce the cost of delivering quality care.

Finally, in a world with an abundance of physician shortages, mHealth will almost certainly expand patient access to all types of care, enabling remote monitoring of chronic conditions, creating new mobile apps, offering 24/7 virtual "office" visits, and gathering medical specialists "in the same room" for more accurate diagnoses and treatment plans.

Around the globe, the mHealth revolution is well under way. As you read through this book, you will learn about the progress and challenges in the mHealth world, as well as gain some insights from important lessons learned. I encourage you to think beyond the four walls of the hospital, not only when reading this book but throughout your journey to transform health care.

Geeta Nayyar, M.D., MBA
Chief Medical Information Officer
PatientPoint

Introduction

Why did we write a book on mobile health (mHealth)? Because we believe it is an essential tool in the disruptive transformation required to change our healthcare system from one that is driven by volume to one that is sustained on value.

Although medicine, with its powerful imaging machines, robotic surgeons, and electronic monitors and devices, is one of the most technology-heavy industries in the world, it lags far behind most other industries when it comes to harnessing the power of *information* technology. This is particularly true when it comes to using that technology to enhance the patient experience, track and improve quality, and manage and reduce costs.

It is still one of the few industries in which data is more likely to be transmitted via fax machine than computer; where records are filed on metal shelves rather than in the cloud; and where the end user—the patient—is often treated as an afterthought rather than the center of the process.

Banking, airlines, transportation, shopping—all have been dramatically transformed by mobile technology and wireless communication in the past five years, with paradigm shifts in how businesses and customers interact and, indeed, how they do business overall. From snapping a photo of a check to deposit it to using the phone as digital currency to purchase a cappuccino, mobile is not just mobile cellular, but *mobile living*.

Now juxtapose these experiences with those of health care. Your doctor might have your health information in an electronic record, but can you get to your information when you are traveling? Can you schedule an appointment online the same way you schedule a restaurant reservation? Can you enter your daily blood pressure so it automatically links to your central health record and alerts a clinician if something's wrong?

Probably not.

We need mHealth to enhance the patient experience and to help us manage the out-of-control costs of modern medicine. In 2011, it cost more than $20,000 to provide health care for the average insured family in the United States—nearly a seven percent increase over 2011. That's more than *three times* the inflation rate for that year. These spiraling increases are unsustainable. They contributed to the bankruptcy of the U.S. auto industry and, if allowed to continue unchecked, will bankrupt the United States and other countries throughout the world.

As we highlight later in the book, if we don't reign in costs, by 2021 health care will make up nearly one-fifth of the U.S. gross domestic product (GDP), a 9.5 percent increase from 17.9 percent in 2009. Data from the Organisation for Economic Co-operation and Development (OECD) finds the United States is not alone when it comes to rapidly increasing healthcare costs. Japan, Britain, Switzerland, and Spain, among others, face the same financial cliff.

We're already recognizing substantial savings with mHealth. Here are just a few examples from across the globe:

- Remotely monitoring heart failure patients after discharge led to a six percent readmission rate compared to the 47 percent national average.

- Remotely monitoring fetal heart rate in women with high-risk pregnancies reduced hospitalizations and outpatient visits.

- Using telehealth to monitor 3,230 people with diabetes, chronic obstructive pulmonary disease, or heart failure for a year led to an 18 percent drop in emergency hospital admissions, a 44 percent drop in deaths, and shorter hospital stays, with no increase in costs.

- Using mHealth to provide follow-up care after the initial diagnosis and treatment of atopic dermatitis found similar outcomes to usual care, but significantly lower costs. Researchers estimated an annual savings in direct and indirect costs (such as absenteeism) of $943 per patient in the first year.

In the developing world, mHealth is needed not to *transform* healthcare systems, but to *develop* the systems in countries with little infrastructure. That's why, as you'll see later in the book, the developing world is using the availability of faster, cheaper, more reliable, interoperable technology, particularly that available through cellular phones and tablets, to bring health care to millions of people without the need to build hospitals or clinics.

mHealth applications have significant relevance in other areas of healthcare reform, including reducing complication rates, emergency department visits, and hospital admissions; improving outcomes through better tracking and monitoring; realizing the goals of population-based preventive care; and enhancing patient involvement and engagement.

However, several daunting challenges exist, particularly around the twin issues of privacy and security. There is also a need for better stewardship of the data that is flowing between patient and caregiver. Overcoming those barriers is critical if mHealth is to reach its full potential.

Our work on this book convinces us that coupling mHealth to the twin engines of electronic health records and healthcare reform is vital if we are to experience the kind of fundamental changes in healthcare delivery required in the United States and other countries. It is also, we are certain, the only way to deliver health care in the developing world, where there may be a single doctor for 10,000 people, and where the majority of medical services are provided not by physicians or nurses, but by community health workers with little access to transportation, electricity, or hospitals.

As the Institute of Medicine wrote in its 2012 report, *Best Care at Lower Cost*, mobile technologies have the potential to substantially change the way health care is delivered and consumed. We could not agree more.

And, as you will see in the pages that follow, the revolution has already started.

Chapter 1. mHealth: The Coming Revolution

"At the end of the day, mHealth is not about smartphones, gadgets, or even apps. It's about holistically driving transformation ... about distributing care beyond clinics and hospitals and enabling new information-rich relationships between patients, clinicians, and caregivers to drive better decisions and behaviors."

Rick Cnossen, Director of Worldwide Health Information Technology, Intel,

Speaking at the 2011 mHealth Congress[1]

Martha, a 66-year-old systems analyst who loves to garden and hike, just had her left knee replaced. She knew she'd need physical therapy when she left the hospital. But there was one thing she didn't know she'd be getting: a tiny sensor weighing less than an ounce to wear behind her ear. The sensor is designed to capture how often and how well she walks, wirelessly transmitting the data to her electronic health record and alerting her doctor of any problems. This enables the doctor to monitor and track the progress of her physical therapy as well as identify any potentially risky problems, such as infection or implant failure, before they become serious.

The scene described above is not taken from science fiction, but from an actual clinical trial.[2] It represents the fastest-growing arena in information technology, one with the potential to transform how health care is delivered in the tiniest, most isolated villages in sub-Saharan Africa or the gleaming "medicalopolises" of New York City, Los Angeles, and Boston. It's already changing how we practice medicine here at the Cleveland Clinic.

We're talking about mobile health, or mHealth, a technological revolution built on the foundation of today's wireless technology, ubiquitous broadband access, and deep market penetration of smartphones and tablets. We call it "Pervasive Health Information Technology," or pHIT (pronounced "fit"), a phrase we created to describe the devices, sensors, and connectivity that will soon be pervasive throughout health care and that will fundamentally reshape the way such care is delivered

mHealth Defined

So just what *is* mHealth? Depends on whom you ask.

The Health Information and Management Systems Society (HIMSS) collected the following definitions from various mHealth-related entities:[3]

Foundation for the National Institutes of Health: "mHealth is the delivery of healthcare services via mobile communication devices."

National Institutes of Health Consensus Group: "mHealth is the use of mobile and wireless devices to improve health outcomes, healthcare services and health research."

mHealth Alliance: "mHealth stands for mobile-based or mobile-

mHealth Defined

enhanced solutions that deliver health. The ubiquity of mobile devices in the developed or developing world presents the opportunity to improve health outcomes through the delivery of innovative medical and health services with information and communication technologies to the farthest reaches of the globe."

The National Broadband Plan: "The use of mobile networks and devices in supporting e-care. Emphasizes leveraging health-focused applications on general-purpose tools such as smartphones and short message service (SMS) messaging to drive active health participation by consumers and clinicians."

West Wireless Health: "The delivery of health care services via mobile communication devices such as cell phones. Applications range from targeted text messages to promote healthy behavior to wide-scale alerts about disease outbreaks. The proliferation of cell phones across the globe, even in locales without basic health care infrastructure, is spurring the growth of mHealth in developing countries."

World Health Organization: "The provision of health services and information via mobile technologies such as mobile phones and personal digital assistants (PDAs)."[4]

Our definition? All of these and more.

mHealth includes everything from that knee sensor to apps that measure and transmit blood pressure and oxygenation levels, enabling imaging results to be read on a tablet or smartphone. It is electronic health records (EHR) that patients and physicians access from their phones, embedded devices that monitor defibrillators and other implantable devices for malfunction, and smartphones that can perform ultrasounds and electrocardiograms.

mHealth is healthcare providers texting appointment and medication reminders to patients, and patients texting blood pressure readings and pain ratings to providers. It's typing the phrase "ER" into a smartphone and getting a text message that lists waiting times at local emergency rooms *and* lets you preregister.

mHealth is secure email between clinicians and patients; radiologists reading MRI images on their iPads; and neurologists assessing stroke in patients hundreds of miles away to determine if they should receive lifesaving, clot-busting drugs.

At its core, mHealth is a new way of interacting with patients that is divorced from the traditional "four-walls-and-an-examining-table" model. It's the ability to provide care over a multitude of media without being physically present.

Most significantly, the "virtual health assistants" that mHealth makes possible shift the focus of health care from episodic "sick" visits to one of continuity and health maintenance. This shift, in turn, has the potential to drive wellness, reduce disease, improve medication compliance, and reduce costs.

Way Cool: Skyping Ultrasounds

In Canada, pulmonologists are assessing patients hundreds of miles away for apnea and pneumothorax using ultrasound performed by people with little or no experience with the technology. The images are streamed via Skype on an iPhone to the doctors, who direct the test remotely.

The procedure has been used for patients in two remote mountain sites, a small airplane in flight, and a household in Calgary with the doctors located in Pisa or Rome, Italy, Philadelphia, or Calgary. All 20 cases had excellent results.

Way Cool: Skyping Ultrasounds

Other clinicians are using similar technology to image patients during trauma, perform fetal wellness assessments, and evaluate vascular anatomy.[5]

Mobile health is not new. Ever since someone sent the first telegram with test results on a patient or held the first phone consult, we've been using mobile health applications. What *is* new is that for the first time we can reach nearly all humans on the planet with health information and monitor their health remotely, opening the potential for a dramatic shift in how we think about health and deliver medical care.

The reality is that we are "virtualizing" the healthcare system overall, and mobile health is a subset of that larger shift. The ultimate goal? To remove time and space as barriers to health care.

What's Going on Out There?

Despite the rapid growth of mHealth throughout health care, we're still learning how individual organizations have integrated the technology into their institutions. The second annual HIMSS Mobile Technology Survey conducted in 2012, surveyed 180 respondents about how their organizations were using mHealth. Fifty-two percent said they thought the use of mobile technology would substantially impact the delivery of health care in the future.[6]

Other pertinent findings:

- ✓ Ninety-three percent reported that physicians used mobile technology during their daily activities, with 80 percent using mobile technology to provide patient care.
- ✓ About two thirds reported that clinicians at their organization either viewed patient information using an app or looked up non-protected health information on a mobile device.
- ✓ Just 22 percent said that all the data captured by mobile devices was integrated into the organization's electronic health record (EHR).
- ✓ Respondents overall characterized their mobile environments as "average" in terms of overall maturity.
- ✓ Sixty-eight percent reported that their organization had a mobile technology plan in place, up from the 38 percent of in 2011. Another third said their organization was developing one.
- ✓ Slightly more than a third (36 percent) allowed patients/consumers to access their medication information via mobile devices.
- ✓ Just 13 percent were developing apps for patients.

Obviously, there is significant room for growth in the use of mobile technology in health care, particularly when it comes to integrating the data collected via apps into the all-important EHR. After all, if we can't do that, we can't use this information to improve clinical care.

Respondents said the key benefits of mobile technology was improved access to patient information and the ability to view data from a remote location, while the main barriers were lack of funding and security concerns.

You'll read more about how healthcare providers are integrating mHealth into their practices and institutions in Chapter 3.

A Perfect Storm

We are all immigrants entering a new country and a new age. Change is coming as we transition from a volume-based health care system to a value-based system, where providers get paid based on the results, quality of care, efficiency, and patient satisfaction.

The tsunami of mHealth is being driven by a perfect storm of out-of-control healthcare costs, a shift from acute-care focus to a focus on chronic and preventive care, and the availability of faster, more reliable, and cheaper interoperable technology that even the poorest people in the remotest parts of the globe can access.

In developed countries like the United States, it's also being driven by patients. Today's patients want to be equal partners in their health care. Thus, they are rejecting the traditional paternalistic doctor-patient relationship.

The tsunami is also being driven by the size and strength of the healthcare industry.

The end result is a global industry expected to reach $26 billion in revenues by 2017.[7] Even that prediction is likely low, given some estimates that put global mHealth revenues in 2012 at $1.5 trillion.[8] Between 2010 and 2015, experts predict the industry will grow between 12 percent and 16 percent.[9]

The U.S. patient monitoring market alone, which includes hospital-based hardware such as wireless ambulatory telemetry monitors and low-tech apps and sensors to monitor chronic conditions, is estimated to grow 35.5 percent, from $3.1 billion in 2011 to nearly $4.2 billion by 2018.[10] Just the health sensor market alone will hit $5.6 billion globally by 2017 compared to $407 million in 2012, predicted German-based research firm research2guidance in 2013.[11]

Indeed, industry analysts predict that the growth of mHealth in the near future will rival that of the Internet in the 1990s. They foresee the fastest growth in home and disease management monitoring; remote physician services such as video consultation; personal emergency services that automatically transmit data to the emergency room for heart attacks or other medical crises; video diagnostic consultations with patients; and remote cardiac services like those that wirelessly transmit a record of defibrillator shocks.[12]

Already, iTunes offers more than 12,000 health-related applications, while a Google search on mobile health care in late 2012 brought up 1.67 million results. Compare that to 5,000 hits in 2007.[1,13]

If that's not a sign of a revolution, then what is?

Unfortunately, the healthcare industry has been slow to join the revolution. As U.S. Health and Human Services (HHS) Secretary Kathleen Sebelius said during the 2011 mHealth Congress: "Over the last few decades, we've seen information technology improve the consumer experience in almost every area of our lives. We've gone from waiting until a bank opened to make a deposit to 24-hour ATMs and paying bills online. But health care has stubbornly held onto its cabinets and hanging files."[1] And, if we can add to her statement, fax machines.

Yet the sheer size of the U.S. healthcare industry, the depth of its dysfunction, and the significant challenges it faces mean it can no longer pretend it is still 1990.

Cost as a Driver

Cost is one of the biggest drivers for this shift. In 2012, it cost more than $20,000 to provide health care for the average insured family in the United States—a nearly 7 percent increase over 2011[14] That's more than *three times* the inflation rate for that year. These spiraling increases are unsustainable. They contributed to the bankruptcy of the U.S. auto industry and, if allowed to continue unchecked, will bankrupt the United States and other countries throughout the world.

"The one clearly bipartisan agenda in Washington is the management of value (in health care)," says Chief Information Officer at the Cleveland Clinic C. Martin Harris, M.D. The issue is crucial, he says, because even if you flatten the inflation curve, sheer volume from an aging population will continue to drive Medicare costs to unsustainable levels. mHealth offers an opportunity to slow the growth in spending by providing an important tool for restructuring the healthcare system.

"One of the most cost-effective places to deliver effective health care is in the home, community, workplace—any other place than where we have traditionally delivered such care." mHealth provides the ability to get the care into those settings.

Globally, underdeveloped countries are looking to mHealth to provide a cost-effective option for building a healthcare infrastructure in settings where there may be just one hospital for 100,000 people in a 100-mile radius.

And European countries need the cost-savings potential of mHealth if they are to maintain their single-payer health systems in the face of aging populations.

If we don't rein in costs, the Centers for Disease Control and Prevention (CDC) estimates that by 2021 health care will make up nearly one-fifth of the U.S. gross domestic product (GDP) , a 9.5 percent increase from 17.9 percent in 2009. Figures 1-1 and 1-2 depict health care as a percentage of GDP for several Organisation for Economic Co-operation and Development (OECD) countries. It's clear from the data that the United States is not alone when it comes to rapidly increasing healthcare costs.

Figure 1-1. Health Expenditures as a Share of GDP, OECD Countries, 2011

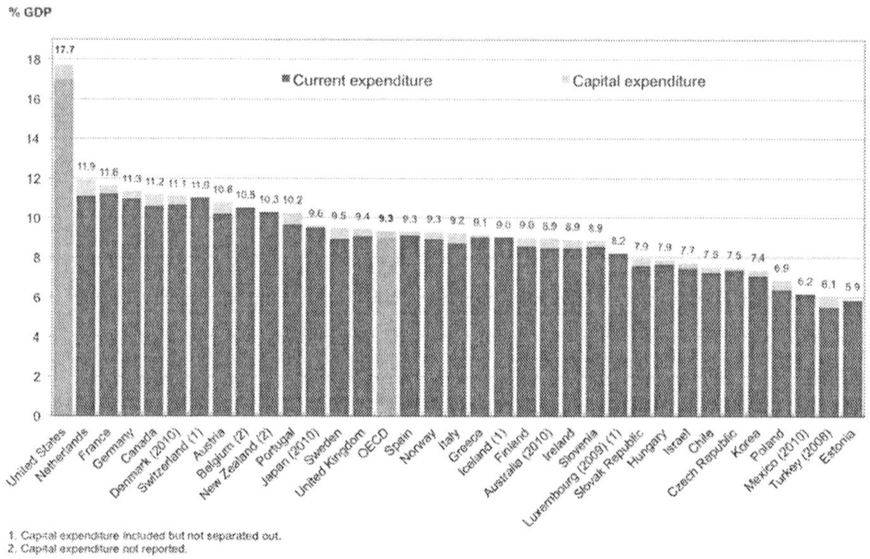

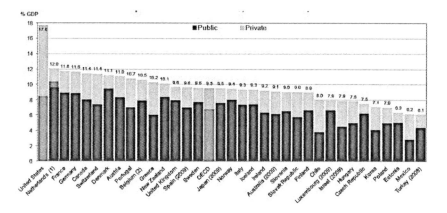

Source: OECD HealthData 2013. How Does the United States Compare.
http://www.oecd.org/unitedstates/Briefing-Note-USA-2013.pdf

Figure 1-2. Total Expenditures, OECD Countries, 2011

Source: OECD HealthData 2013. How Does the United States Compare.
http://www.oecd.org/unitedstates/Briefing-Note-USA-2013.pdf

Thus, there is a huge potential for anything that can shave even a few percentage points off the healthcare bill in the United States and other countries. That's where mHealth comes in.

University of Oxford Professor Lionel Tarassenko estimates that mHealth could save Great Britain's National Health Service £750 million ($1.1 billion) a year by reducing hospital admissions,[15] while Juniper Research's 2010 Mobile Healthcare Opportunities report estimates that just the use of remote patient monitoring via cellular networks could save between $1.96 billion and $5.83 billion in healthcare costs by 2014, most of that in the United States and Canada.[16]

Meanwhile, the consulting firm Accenture predicted in a 2012 analysis that mobile solutions could save the United States more than $23 billion by targeting patients with chronic diseases like diabetes and heart disease, an expected $2,000 to $3,000 per year in savings per disease, per member. Those savings will come from 15 percent to 20 percent fewer hospital days, 30 percent fewer emergency room visits, improved patient outcomes, and more efficient, timely action.[17]

A 2012 research report from the Telenor Group estimates that mHealth could slash medical costs by a quarter among those 65 and older.[18] That same year, the Brookings Institution predicted remote monitoring devices alone could save nearly $200 billion in healthcare costs over the next 25 years.[19]

"With around-the-clock monitoring and electronic data transmission to caregivers, remote devices speed up the treatment of patients requiring medical intervention," the Brookings Institution report noted. "Rather than having to wait for a patient to discover there is a problem, monitors identify deteriorating conditions in real time and alert physicians."[19]

We highlight numerous examples of mHealth savings throughout this book. Here are just a few from hospitals and healthcare systems around the country to whet your appetite:

- Remotely monitoring heart failure patients after discharge led to a 6 percent readmission rate compared to the 47 percent national average.[20]

- Remotely monitoring fetal heart rate in women with high-risk pregnancies reduced hospitalizations and outpatient visits.[21]

- Using digital cameras to document pressure sores in patients and transmit the images to specialists for remote consultations reduced emergency room visits and hospitalizations.[22]

- Using telehealth to monitor 3,230 people with diabetes, chronic obstructive pulmonary disease, or heart failure for a year led to an 18 percent drop in emergency hospital admissions, a 44 percent drop in deaths, and shorter hospital stays, with no increase in costs.[23]

- Using telehealth to provide follow-up care after the initial diagnosis and treatment of atopic dermatitis found similar outcomes to usual care, but significantly lower costs. Researchers estimated an annual savings in direct and indirect costs (such as absenteeism) of $943 per patient in the first year.[24]

Way Cool: Quicker Cardiac Care

When patients with implanted defibrillators and other cardiac devices come into the emergency room, a staff member has to call the device company and wait for a representative to come to the hospital and check the device before the patient can be treated, wasting valuable time and money. A Medtronic device called CareLink Express enables emergency room staff to wirelessly transmit the data to a company representative who assesses the device status. A 50-site pilot program over five months found that hospitals using the system cut the average 84-minute wait time to less than 15 minutes, with one hospital reporting cost savings of nearly $130,000 in less than three months. The CareLink network currently serves more than 6,600 clinics and 720,000 patients in 33 countries.[25]

Payers Want (and Need) mHealth

Health care in the United States and elsewhere is shifting from a volume-based system, in which providers are paid based on what they do rather than on how well they do it, to a value-based system, in which they are paid based on the quality and outcomes of the care provided.

With this shift come incentives for payers to embrace—and pay for—mHealth as a means of reducing costs and improving quality.

Insurers, including the federal government, are slowly recognizing that it makes more sense to incur a one-time $500 cost for an iPad to help patients with diabetes better manage their condition than it does to pay to manage long-term complications like kidney failure and amputations that can occur if the disease is poorly managed.

So, for instance, in 2012 the U.S. Department of Veterans Affairs (VA) announced it would waive patient copayments for in-home video telemonitoring as an incentive to increase the use of such technology.[26] Several health insurers, including WellPoint, Aetna, and Humana, are piloting payment programs for remote monitoring to cut readmissions.[27]

You'll read more about the implications and involvement of payers—both commercial and government—in Chapter 5.

Changing Demographics, Changing Expectations

Aging Baby Boomers are already behaving differently from any other 50- and 60-something demographic we've seen in the past. The "me" generation has always demanded that the market meet *its* demands, not the other way around. Plus, the boomers, their children, and their grandchildren, have grown up in a world of technology.

Way Cool: Belly Band

Researchers from the engineering and media arts schools of Drexel University designed the Belly Band, which contains conductive yarn and an embedded antenna that allows remote monitoring of pregnant patients. The noninvasive band, which does not require batteries or electricity, transmits radio signals to indicate changes in the shape of the uterus and could alert obstetricians to possible pregnancy complications.

They expect instant access to data, demand transparency in their interactions, and insist on playing an active role in major events in their lives. For instance, when we surveyed the population around Cleveland, Ohio, to better understand what people wanted in a primary care provider, it wasn't pedigree, gender, or experience; it was access to their medical records and the ability to interact with their care providers electronically.

Way Cool: Calling in Your Heart Rate

AliveCor has developed a clinical-quality, low-cost mobile ECG heart monitor that fits onto the iPhone and allows patients to monitor their heart health anywhere and anytime.

Most industries—with the exception of health care—have evolved to meet these demands. Consider banks. From ATMs to online banking to deposits via smartphones, the banking industry has taken advantage of new technologies to improve quality and reduce costs. As a result, many consumers haven't set foot in a bank for years.

Aside from meeting the needs of consumers, these mobile transactions have substantial cost savings for businesses. Just consider what the airline industry has accomplished with digitization. These days, it's the customer who does the work, researching flights, booking the flight, purchasing the ticket—even printing out the boarding pass and choosing a seat. Yet, very few healthcare consumers can book an appointment with their physician online, let alone provide basic information like their health history, medications, or even physical address.

Given that we live more and more of our lives online (many of us don't even work in offices any more)[28] why do we have to call our doctor for an appointment, wait a day or more before we're seen, take time off from work, and fight traffic to get to the office, only to wait an hour and be told the doctor can't figure anything out until we get some tests. Couldn't that have been determined via email or Skype?

Indeed, evidence shows that video visits, Skyping, and even emailing providers can dramatically improve access to care for home-bound, frail elderly, or disabled individuals, as well as significantly increase access for people living in underserved rural areas in the United States and other countries.[29] If it works for these populations, we figure it will work for younger, healthier, more urban populations, as well. Music, books, television programs, and movies—all available with a few clicks when and where we want them. So, why not health care? That's the questions consumers are asking.

Beyond the convenience and transparency, consumers want mHealth because they expect it to improve the cost of care.[30] They need it. Today, healthcare consumers pay more out of pocket in deductibles, copayments, and coinsurances than ever before, prompting them for the first time to ask: "How much will it cost?" Show them that a $50 home blood glucose monitor that wirelessly feeds data to their EHR can help them improve their glucose control and, consequently, save $100 a month in drug costs, and you've got yourself a sale.

We'll cover the patient aspect of the mHealth revolution in more detail in Chapter 4.

"Connectivity between and across patients and health systems promises to be one of the most important advances that can enable a more distributed form of healthcare delivery at a lower cost"

Rank J.
Mobile Operators and Digital Health. 2012.

The Technological Revolution

Just as the availability of the Internet, Facebook, Twitter, and smartphones propelled revolutions in Tunisia, Egypt, Libya, and Yemen during the so-called Arab Spring in 2011, so, too, are these components driving the mHealth revolution, particularly in underdeveloped and undeveloped countries.

Consider that there were an estimated *6 billion* cellphones in use as of 2012, with an astounding 86 percent of the world's population subscribed to a cellular service.[31] A survey that year from the Pew Research Internet & American Life Project found that 85 percent of adults in the United States owned cellphones, half of them smartphones. The survey also found that a third of cellphone users used their devices to research health or medical information online, with Hispanics the greatest users. This is particularly relevant given the growth of the Hispanic demographic as a percentage of the overall population.[32]

The survey also found plenty of room for growth, given that just 19 percent of smartphone users had downloaded a health-based app and just 9 percent receive health-related text messages.

Plus, there is a relatively low barrier to entry for many mHealth applications. After all, you can develop an app these days for less than $100. This is, as you'll see later, both a blessing and a curse.

Case Study: Diabetes and mHealth

An estimated one out of 10 adults in the United States has diabetes, which is the seventh leading cause of death for Americans.[33,34] By 2050, unless we make behavioral changes, one in three Americans will have diabetes.[35] Globally, 366 million people have diabetes; by 2030, that figure will nearly double.[36]

Given the staggeringly high costs of the global diabetes epidemic ($465 billion in 2011 to treat diabetes and prevent complications) and the disease's high morbidity and mortality rates, these projections are, quite simply, frightening.[2]

So, finding ways to improve care and reduce costs for people with diabetes is critical.

Enter mHealth.

According to the eHealth Initiative, a nonprofit organization that researches and identifies ways to use information technology to improve the quality, safety, and efficiency of health care, mobile health technology can improve diabetes control and reduce healthcare spending for patients, regardless of their socioeconomic status.[37] The technology studied included patient portals that integrate EHRs and patient health records and allow secure messaging between patients and providers, and social media sites that allow patients to share their experiences.

Among the examples the organization highlighted in a 2012 report sponsored by the California HealthCare Foundation:[37]

WellDoc Diabetes Manager System. This mobile health

Case Study: Diabetes and mHealth

application uses real-time data such as blood glucose values and diet to provide automated weekly coaching. In a one-year, randomized controlled trial, 150 people using the system in conjunction with a glucose monitor significantly reduced their blood glucose levels.

DiaBetNet. This wireless personal digital assistant uses a motivational game to help kids between 8 and 18 manage their type 2 diabetes. Participants in a six-month pilot study significantly improved their overall knowledge of diabetes and blood glucose levels.

The iglucose Mobile Health Solution. This program collects and wirelessly transmits data from electronic blood glucose meters to a diabetes management portal where it can be shared with healthcare professionals. The tool includes reports to track health and communicate between clinicians and patients.

You'll read more about mHealth and diabetes throughout the book.

Oh Where, Oh Where Have All the Doctors Gone?

The looming physician shortage in the United States and elsewhere in the world increases the need for mHealth. In the United States, the expected influx of 30 million newly insured individuals into the healthcare system in 2014 has spurred a plethora of dire predictions about a gridlocked system. Medicare and Medicaid patients already have trouble finding doctors. The aging boomers— who will require more medical care—and the more than 30 million previously uninsured Americans who will enter the system in 2014 will exacerbate that problem.

Obviously, we can't suddenly train 10,000 new doctors. And with reimbursement as low as it is (and facing more cuts in the near future), it is challenging to convince medical school students to specialize in relatively lower-paying fields like family medicine, internal medicine, and pediatrics—areas where they are most needed.

Enter technology. We can harness the power of mobile health to allow clinicians to work smarter, rather than harder, and to care for more patients with no loss in quality. We're already doing it. Just consider the remote intensive care unit, in which clinicians at a central station remotely monitor more than a dozen patients at once, much like air traffic controllers tracking multiple jets. Unlike an air traffic controller, however, physicians can provide some of this oversight even when off site thanks to data streaming into a tablet or smartphone and video monitoring.

In fact, research from PwC found that 56 percent of physicians who use mobile devices in their practices say they can make decisions more quickly, and 40 percent say they spend less time on administrative tasks (Figure 1-3).[30] As the report noted: "Such shifts could rewrite physician supply and shortage forecasts for the next decade and beyond."[30]

Figure 1-3. Physician Expectations of mHealth

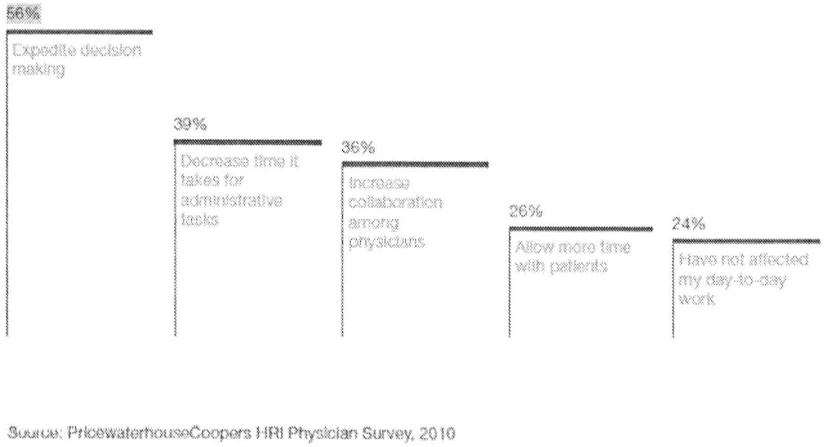

56%
Expedite decision making

39%
Decrease time it takes for administrative tasks

36%
Increase collaboration among physicians

26%
Allow more time with patients

24%
Have not affected my day-to-day work

Source: PricewaterhouseCoopers HRI Physician Survey, 2010

As healthcare reform drives practice change, we are also entering the realm of *population health*. No longer can we focus just on the individual; we need to shift to a proactive and participatory collaboration with a population. That population might be defined by a disease, a procedure, or a treatment, or it might be a cohort of patients who are focused on stress reduction and wellness. Regardless, mHealth can play a crucial role in identifying, engaging, and uniting healthcare providers in their quest to improve the health of a population.

Picture a physician group responsible for 10,000 patients with diabetes. The group's income is increasingly tied to a slew of quality indicators such as A1C levels, foot and eye exams, and blood pressure medication adherence. How can it ensure it follows practice guidelines and meets treatment goals for 10,000 patients?

Through mHealth, of course.

For instance, the group could run a monthly report highlighting all diabetes patients who need foot exams, automatically send out electronic reminders, track those who make and keep the appointments, and trigger automated telephone call reminders for those who don't. We call this "push technology for chronic care."

At the Federal Level

HHS, as well as numerous other government agencies, sees mHealth as an important way to improve quality and reduce costs. So it is jumping into the mHealth pool with both feet. Among current initiatives:

- The National Cancer Institute's SmokefreeTXT program, a mobile smoking cessation service designed for teens and young adults across the United States.

- A partnership between the Office of Minority Health, the American Association of Diabetes Educators, AT&T, and Baylor University to use smartphones to provide live diabetes self-management education courses, accompanied by text prompts and reminders, in healthcare provider shortage areas.

- A partnership with the White House to launch the Apps Against Abuse challenge, a national competition that calls upon technology developers to create innovative applications to offer young adults a way to connect with trusted friends in real-time to prevent abuse or violence.

- An mHealth community of practice, open to all HHS staff, to help evaluate mHealth activities and practices across the department.

Other initiatives include the HHS text4baby program to improve prenatal and first-year health, the Text Alert Toolkit for emergency response, and the Text4Health program, charged with developing recommendations for mHealth technology that has the potential to improve health.[38]

The Federal Communications Commission (FCC) has been preparing for the mHealth revolution for years. In 2010, it issued the country's first National Broadband Plan, which identified health care as an area of "enormous promise for broadband-enabled innovation." The plan includes a chapter of recommendations on health care and led to a partnership between the FCC and the U.S. Food and Drug Administration (FDA) to "help ensure that communications-related medical innovations can swiftly and safely be brought to market."

In November 2011, the FCC dedicated spectrum for Medical Micro-Power Networks, an ultra-low–power wideband network consisting of a MedRadio programmer/control transmitter and medical implant transmitters that transmit or receive non-voice data or related device control commands to enable functional electric stimulation. This technique uses electric currents to activate and monitor nerves and muscles that could, as the agency's chair Julius Genachowski noted, "enable paraplegics to stand and restore sight to the blind." The regulation made the United States the first country in the world to devote bandwidth to this technology.

In 2012, the FCC issued a 26-page report on the findings of its mHealth task force, outlining five recommendations:[39]

1. The FCC should continue to play a leadership role in advancing mobile health adoption.

2. Federal agencies should increase collaboration to promote innovation, protect patient safety, and avoid regulatory duplication.

3. The FCC should build on existing programs and link programs where possible to expand broadband access for health care.

4. The FCC should continue efforts to increase capacity, reliability, interoperability, and radio frequency safety of mHealth technologies.

5. Industry should support continued investment, innovation, and job creation in the growing mHealth sector.

Genachowski announced that the agency would implement all recommendations and would recruit a permanent director to work with external groups on all health-related issues.

Barriers to mHealth

Nothing comes easily in health care, and mHealth is no different. We cover barriers to successful mHealth integration throughout the book, focusing on security and privacy in Chapter 2. We want to preview several here.

Privacy. This is perhaps the biggest elephant in the room when it comes to mHealth barriers. All medical applications and interactions between healthcare providers and physicians must adhere to HIPAA requirements. That's the federal Health Insurance Portability and Accountability Act, which guarantees patient privacy. The penalties for violating HIPAA rules are steep, so mHealth developers and users have a strong incentive to build privacy protection into all technology.

But with the field so diverse, and so much data hosted in the cloud, it's not clear how this will play out. For instance, what if the manufacturer of a calorie counter app sold its customer list to a grocery store, which then targeted customers with coupons and promotions for low-calorie food? Is that a HIPAA violation?

Security. Beyond the security associated with hacking and/or lost or stolen data, which can lead to HIPAA violations, there is the security of the devices and monitors themselves that form the core of mHealth. We're talking about implantable defibrillators and insulin pumps, sensors like the one described in the opening of this chapter, video streams between clinicians and patients—often using "virtual" tools for diagnosis—and commands sent wirelessly to powerful MRIs and CT scans. What if someone hacks into *those* devices? What kind of havoc could they create?

Technological issues. The global cellular/digital network is better today than even five years ago—but it's not nearly as good or reliable as it must be if we're to practice medicine over it. This is particularly true in the United States, which has a significantly weaker cellular grid than many other countries. Just think about the number of dropped calls, black holes, and "all circuits are busy" signals you get in an average week. That's fine if you're calling to make an appointment with your doctor; not so fine if your doctor is trying to manage a stroke from 200 miles away. Fixing the digital pipes is expensive; who will pay?

Plus, too few systems talk to each other. Although the Cleveland Clinic is fully integrated, with our systems communicating seamlessly (on a good day), but communicating with physicians and healthcare entities that aren't in our system often brings us back to paper and fax.

This lack of interoperability is a huge barrier to digitizing health information and improving care coordination, and it will be a huge barrier to seamlessly integrating mHealth technologies.

Reimbursement. Although, as noted earlier, payers are beginning to provide reimbursement for mHealth technology, most of those efforts are still in the pilot stage. We need wholesale coverage for mHealth costs, both hardware and software, to fully realize its potential.

"The realignment of reimbursement policy for telemedicine is among the most critical requirements."[29]

Rank J.
Mobile Operators and Digital Health. 2012.

Technological relevance. We're concerned about technology developers who fail to keep the end user in mind. For instance, we recently evaluated a program designed to provide discharge planners with quality information and bed availability at nearby skilled nursing and long-term care facilities. What's the point? The discharge planners already know which are the best post-acute facilities, and the facilities themselves keep the planners updated on bed availability. It is important that the technology we ask providers and patients to adopt is relevant and hits the mark right out of the gate.

"Stickiness." We also wonder if patients or providers will continue using the technology once the novelty wears off. After all, how many of us use our gym after January or maintain an online food diary app for more than a week or two?

Data quality. Many of the uses for mHealth rely on reams of data. But you know what they say: "Garbage in, garbage out." How will we evaluate and maintain the integrity of the data and science used for many of the apps and technologies now entering the market? More importantly, how will we mine the reams of data created by sensors, apps, and monitors for that which is truly relevant?

Provider reluctance. You'd think doctors, nurses, healthcare administrators, and others would be thrilled to embrace anything that helps them do their jobs faster and better, with the potential for significant savings. Sadly, you'd be wrong. Although the younger generation of healthcare professionals that grew up with iTunes, Xbox, and laptops is committed to mHealth, the generation before them—which includes many of their bosses, mentors, and teachers—often cling to their paper charts like a drowning man to a life raft.

Older physicians threaten to retire before converting their paper-based offices to digital; many clinicians still prefer to communicate by fax; and even the most wired hospitals hand you a piece of paper when you register. In fact, a PwC survey found that nearly a third of doctors and a third of payers said an "inherently conservative culture" is a leading barrier to mHealth.[30]

Regulation. The variety of government agencies likely to regulate mHealth here and in other countries, coupled with the complexity and heterogeneity of those regulations, provides another potential barrier.

The FDA tried to regulate digital devices and software before. In 1989, with the use of computer and software products in the medical field growing exponentially, it issued its "Draft Software Policy." However, as the number of devices and programs continued to explode, the FDA determined that "it would be impractical to prepare an overarching software policy to address all of the issues related to the regulation of all medical devices containing software," and it withdrew the policy.

Since then, its main role has been to approve software used to analyze medical device data when used as part of that device. This is the kind of authority that enabled it to approve a mobile radiology app so physicians could view medical images on iPhones and iPads. In the past couple of years, the FDA has also been dipping its toe into the medical app arena, approving a handful of apps and devices such as an opthalmoscope device that plugs into a smart phone and, together with the attendant app, enables clinicians to diagnose conditions like retinal detachment or glaucoma; a device that turns an iPhone into an electrocardiogram recorder; and an app that enables clinicians to share any kind of digital images.

Since then, the FDA has issued proposed outlines for its role in regulating the world of mHealth and has promised final rules by the end of 2013 on an "appropriate, risk-based regulatory framework pertaining to health information technology, including mobile medical applications, that promotes innovation, protects patient safety, and avoids regulatory duplication."

How that will work is anyone's guess, given that the agency currently takes about six months to approve a medical device similar to an existing product and 20 months to approve a brand-new device. Superimposing that on an mHealth world in which an app can enter the market in January and be obsolete by May seems difficult to imagine.

Top Paid Medical Apps for iPhones[40]

USA Today listed the following as the top medical apps for iPhones sold in the iTunes store in 2011. While the list has likely changed by now, it gives you a good sense of what's popular. It's also interesting to note that half are for healthcare providers—an indication of the potential demand from medical professionals for new ways of obtaining information.

1. **Pill Identifier.** Allows you to identify more than 10,000 over-the-counter and prescription pills based on their appearance.

2. **Pregnancy ++.** Tracks the course of a pregnancy, including the woman's weight, diet, and exercise. Even includes sonogram pictures, a "kick counter," and a contraction counter.

3. **Baby Connect.** Tracks a baby's everyday activities (including feeding, sleep, growth, health, and vaccines) and creates graphical reports and trending charts that can be shared with others.

4. **Instant ECG.** Uses video demonstrations of more than 30 arrhythmias to teach healthcare professionals the basics of reading electrocardiograms (ECGs).

5. **MedCalc.** Provides more than 200 diagnostic formulas, scores, scales, and classifications to help clinicians measure overall health.

6. **Pill Reminder.** Tracks medications, vitamins, and supplements; provides reminders to take and refill medications; and checks for drug interactions, dosage information, and possible side effects.

7. **Anatomy 3D: Organs.** Uses 3D models, videos, audio lectures, diagrams, quizzes, and a glossary to teach anatomy.

8. **Diagnosaurus DDx.** It's a little scary to think of your doctor using an app to figure out what's wrong with you, but that's exactly what Diagnosaurus DDx does. The doctor can search more than 1,000 diagnoses by organ system, symptom, and disease, and use a special feature to consider alternative diagnoses when multiple conditions are possible.

Top Paid Medical Apps for iPhones[40]

9. **Everyday First Aid**. Uses American Red Cross guidelines to show how to handle emergencies such as choking, wound cleaning, jellyfish stings, tick bites, and heart attacks. (Note: If someone is choking or having a heart attack, call 911 before searching an app.)

10. **Drugs & Bugs**. Offers information on more than 100 antibiotics and nearly 200 bacterial pathogens, enabling clinicians to compare the effectiveness of various drugs.

Moving Forward

Can You Imagine ...

In 2012, Google released Google Glass, eyeglasses with an integrated computer and camera. Imagine their potential in health care! That's just what several people did in responding to a blog about the topic. They suggested the glasses could be used to:

✓ Superimpose a labeled overlay onto the cadaver in the anatomy lab, with the labels changing with head movement.

✓ Enable radiologists to read imaging studies without a computer, tablet, or smartphone.

✓ Allow surgeons to view imaging studies during surgery without shifting their attention from the surgical field to peer at a film or computer.

✓ Enable patients to look down any street and interact with

Can You Imagine ...

providers in that area, viewing availability, pricing, the doctor's ratings on Angie's List, and the insurances they accept.

✓ Maintain eye contact with patients and colleagues while simultaneously pulling up information on a disease state.

So yes, there are several challenges facing mHealth, some of which may, at times, feel insurmountable. But as you'll see throughout the rest of this book, organizations, institutions, and governments *are* finding ways to overcome those barriers. They have to. The stakes are just too big.

Chapter 1: Key Takeaways

✓ Devices, sensors, and cellular connectivity will soon be pervasive throughout health care, fundamentally changing the way such care is delivered.

✓ Globally, the mHealth industry is expected to reach $26 billion in revenues by 2017.

✓ The U.S. healthcare industry has been slow to join the mHealth revolution.

✓ Major drivers of mHealth include out-of-control healthcare costs, a shift from an acute-care to a chronic- and preventive-care medical system and from a fee-for-service to a value-based reimbursement system, the need for greater quality and coordinated care, and more reliable and cheaper interoperable technology that even the poorest people in the remotest parts of the globe can access.

✓ mHealth is already demonstrating significant cost savings.

✓ Several barriers to the successful implementation of mHealth exist, including security and privacy issues, institutional culture, technological challenges, and reimbursement.

Chapter 2. Privacy and Security—The Elephant in the Room

"I have never seen an industry with more gaping security holes [than the healthcare industry]. If our financial industry regarded security the way the health-care sector does, I would stuff my cash in a mattress under my bed."

Avi Rubin,
Computer Scientist and Technical Director of the Information Security Institute at Johns Hopkins University, in a 2012 interview with *The Washington Post*[41]

Think you've done enough to protect your wireless systems, apps, and devices? Then consider:

- In Libertyville, Ill., a surgical practice was hacked, and the hacker posted a message on the practice's server saying the contents had been encrypted and could only be accessed with a password—which the hackers would provide for a ransom. The breach affected the data of more than 7,000 patients.[42]

- In Palo Alto, Calif., a hospital reported an unencrypted laptop stolen from a physician's car. The laptop contained information about 57,000 patients.[43]

- Between 2009 and 2011, the U.S. Department of Veterans Affairs (VA) reported 173 incidents of security breaches that disrupted glucose monitors, canceled patient appointments, and shut down sleep labs. In addition, the VA reported in March 2013 that it had transmitted unencrypted health data between medical centers and community-based outpatient clinics.[44]

- The Centers for Medicare and Medicaid Services (CMS) tracks nearly 300,000 compromised Medicare-beneficiary numbers.[8]

- The Office for Civil Rights has received more than 77,000 complaints regarding breaches of health information privacy and completed more than 27,000 investigations, resulting in more than 18,000 corrective actions.[8]

- Government auditors from the Office of Inspector General of the Department of Health and Human Services (HHS) demonstrated that it was possible to obtain patient information from unsecured hospital wireless networks while sitting in the hospital parking lot with a laptop.[8]

Hackers broke into a network server at the Utah Health Department in March 2012, gained access to Medicaid data about 780,000 people, and stole an undetermined number of records. Authorities traced the breach to computers in Eastern Europe.[41]

In the last three years, more than 21 million medical records were exposed—and those are just the security breaches large enough to be reported.[45] You can bet that as mHealth becomes more ubiquitous within medicine, those breaches will reach new heights. As security expert and CEO of Sensato, John Gomez, said in an interview: "Healthcare security is, on average, five years behind other high-tech industries."

The potential repercussions of compromised patient data are significant. The stolen and hacked information can be used for insurance fraud, redirecting valuable financial resources, and putting patients at financial risk. It can also affect the quality of care if the perpetrator changes information in the patient's medical record and could lead to rejections of needed drugs and supplies if the patient's record falsely shows that the patient already received the items.[8] Indeed, half of the 80 healthcare organizations surveyed last year by consulting firm Ponemon Institute reported at least one incident of medical identity theft.[46]

It's About Trust

The greatest threat that breaches of security and privacy pose is their ability to undermine our trust in health information technology and, by extension, the entire healthcare system. This foundation is critical—patients and their families and caregivers *must* trust that the sensitive personal information entered into the system remains safe.

Patients share the most intimate aspects of their lives with us as we work together to improve their health. We have, on more than one occasion, had patients share extremely sensitive information that is critical to their health, information that completely changes our approach to their care. They share that information because they trust us.

This is one reason that caregivers and patients still crave the one-on-one, face-to-face privacy of the exam room. It is a sacred space where crucial conversations are held in strictest confidence. As we move into the world of mHealth, we must be careful to ensure that we protect the trust that lies at the heart of the patient/physician relationship. We need to bring this sacredness to the virtual places we create.

Security and privacy are the two biggest challenges mHealth faces if it is to become more than a few exercise apps on a road warrior's phone. We call them the "elephants in the room," and they are growing before our eyes.

Our own chief integrity officer at Cleveland Clinic, Donald A. Sinko, acknowledges the risks but also notes that there are risks in anything we do. The real challenge is deciding how much risk we are willing to take and what we can do to minimize those risks or mitigate problems when they occur.

"Doctors have to think beyond just protecting patient health to how they can protect patient data." And patients have to understand that when they initiate virtual interactions with healthcare professionals, they are assuming a risk that their email or text message can be hacked and the information stolen, and that it isn't the doctor's fault. You have to know what the risks are and be willing to assume those risks."

At the Cleveland Clinic, which has 44,000 employees, we understand those risks. For instance, just putting the word "Confidential" in the subject line of an email automatically encrypts that email. But it's been a challenge getting our doctors to do that, Sinko said.

Our virus filters capture tens of thousands of attempts *each week* to infiltrate our system. We recently installed sophisticated software called FireEye, which blocks cyber attacks in real time. "We thought we were doing pretty well in this arena until we turned on the software and found that 180 of our computers were infected with malware," Sinko said. The new software also showed us that we get about 20 to 40 previously unrecognized attempts to install malware a week. However, the software is far too expensive for most hospital systems to install, so you can just imagine how many of *their* computers are infected.

Hang On to Your Data

Health care is a "hot new area" for device and data thieves because other industries like banking have become better at thwarting such attempts, says William R. "Bill" Braithwaite, M.D., Ph.D., an original author of the Administrative Simplification Subtitle of the federal Health Insurance Portability and Accountability Act of 1996 (HIPAA) and an expert on the hill and its implementation. "Now the fraudsters that used to go after banks are finding it's much easier and much cheaper to go after medical records," he said, "which still contain all the information necessary to open credit card accounts and bank accounts and rip people off."

> *"Thanks to the rising costs of health care, the value of medical information has skyrocketed in the black markets, making organizations that collect and maintain (personal health information) prime targets for hackers, social engineers, and insiders with malicious intent. Mobilizing all this information makes it a pretty attractive target."*
>
> Mark D. Combs,
> Chief Information Security Officer and Director of Information Technology
> West Virginia University Healthcare, Morgantown

Even scarier are reports of organized crime syndicates embedding people in healthcare organizations to steal data.

How great is the threat? Great enough that the U.S. Department of Homeland Security has expressed fears that activist hackers, cyberwarriors, criminals, and terrorists will attack the healthcare system.[41]

So, it's not surprising that a 2012 report from PwC's Research Institute found that mobile device security is among the top 10 issues facing the healthcare industry this year. Yet, the report found, less than half of hospitals surveyed had a security strategy in place to regulate mobile device use.[30]

That wouldn't surprise Dr. Braithwaite, who says even some chief information officers at hospitals don't understand the concept of multifactor authentication for security. "We have a national effort to improve the care that we provide and to lower its cost by implementing electronic record systems that exchange information," he said. "Yet, we're doing it in such a way that we don't know who is sending the record, who is receiving it, who might have seen it in between, and even who it's about."

Multifactor What?

Multifactor authentication uses two or more factors to establish that *you* are really *you*:

- A *knowledge* factor: something that you know, such as a pin or password.

- A *possession* factor: something currently in your possession, such as an ATM card, phone, or special key fob.

- An *inherence* factor: something that is uniquely part of you; a biometric characteristic, such as a fingerprint or the pattern of arteries and veins in your retina.

These factors can be combined in numerous ways to greatly improve authentication. For example, you might combine tokens that generate a random number that must be used in conjunction

Multifactor What?

with a PIN or password; smartcards that need to be unlocked with a PIN or password; time-limited codes sent via short message service (SMS) in conjunction with a PIN or password; or software-based certificates or credentials stored on the user's device that are accessed via a PIN or password. Any can be combined with or substituted with biometric authentication such as fingerprint or retinal scanning.[47]

Some companies are even experimenting with new forms of authentication that are a cross between biologic and behavioral approaches, such as the patterns in a person's voice or the way they strike the keys of a keyboard.

However, Sinko warns, nothing can be made 100 percent secure with today's technology. Even the U.S. Department of Defense, which you would think is one of the most secure information systems in the world, has been hacked and lost secrets.

Instead, "We need to take very reasonable measures to try and protect our data, knowing we'll never be able to say we're impenetrable," said Sinko.

Ironically, one of the most important barriers to data loss is not some fancy software program, but educating your users, he said.

Security or Privacy?

"Security is what it is; privacy is what you do with the information once you've accessed it in a secure way," said Mary Sirois, principal and clinical transformation practice director at Virginia Beach-based consulting firm Divurgent. "They tie to each other ... they are not completely separate, but they are not joined together, either."

If you haven't figure out what that means for your organization and how you will address each separately and together, then you probably aren't ready to go beyond paper files and locked file cabinets (not that they are always private and secure, either).

As Gomez noted in his presentation during the 2012 mHealth Summit: "The current focus in health information technology is on 'patient privacy' stemming from federal and state HIPAA laws. Privacy compliance is simply about making sure you safeguard the identity of a patient in the event their data is viewed or interacted with by someone the patient did not authorize to view the data. Privacy compliance is kind of cool, but it is totally the wrong thing to be focusing on in this day and age of limited resources and increasing cyber-terrorist threats."

"I tell people that we're very good at keeping information private," he said, "but we have very low concerns about securing our systems so others can't access them."

Bottom line, he said, "Privacy does not always equate to security."

Increasing Breaches

The December 2012 Ponemon report found that the percentage of organizations reporting a breach has increased since the organization began tracking healthcare data breaches in 2010, with more reports of multiple breaches. While 94 percent of the 80 healthcare organizations surveyed had at least one data breach in the past two years, 45 percent had more than five. That compares to 2010, when a third reported more than five. The 2012 survey also found that only 40 percent of companies surveyed felt confident that they could prevent or quickly detect patient data loss or theft.[46]

What's It Costing You?

Between HIPAA fines, lawsuits, and internal investigations, the cost of security and privacy breaches is huge, hitting healthcare systems at a time when many are already operating on thin margins. Ponemon estimates that security breaches cost organizations about $2.5 million over a two-year period, with annual costs to the entire industry of nearly $7 billion.

Look for that amount to rise exponentially given new HIPAA rules that significantly increase fines.

Some companies are even experimenting with new forms of authentication that are a cross between biologic and behavioral approaches, such as the patterns in a person's voice or the way they strike the keys of a keyboard.

Keeping this data safe will only become more difficult as more is held in the cloud and accessed on mobile devices and through file-sharing applications. For instance, in the Ponemon survey, just 9 percent of companies surveyed kept their data out of the cloud. The rest sent it there, even though nearly half reported no confidence in its security. Interestingly, healthcare entities that don't allow their employees to use public file-sharing sites like Dropbox have no problem storing thousands of patient records in the cloud, the report noted.

Another challenge with mobility, notes Sirois, is that someone can walk off and leave their phone (or tablet or laptop) unprotected. "Is the data encrypted?" she asked. "If you lose the device, is there a way of remotely wiping it clean and being able to prove you destroyed that software so if anyone had an issue with it you could prove it wasn't you who leaked the information?" Too often, she says, the answer is "no."

Do You Know the Threats?

- Malware such as worms, viruses, trojan horses, and spyware that can steal data and passwords.

- Eavesdropping on unencrypted data.

- Unauthorized access via stored logins and passwords.

- Theft and loss. One report estimates that Americans lose about $30 billion worth of mobile phones, at least 9 million a year, while about 2.5 billion are lost worldwide. The report estimates that we lose a phone, on average, once a year, and whoever finds the phone is likely to try and access the data.[48] There are apps now that can remotely lock or wipe a phone, including built-in utilities in Apple's iOS and Google's Android operating systems.

- Unlicensed and unmanaged applications that could put a company at legal risk.

By the Numbers

The Ponemon Institute surveyed 80 healthcare organizations and talked to more than 300 managers in late 2012 to assess the state of health information technology privacy and security. Here are some of the top-line findings:[46]

- Each organization had an average of four data breaches in the past two years.

- The average economic impact of a data breach over the past two years for these organizations was $2.4 million.

By the Numbers

- An average of 2,769 records were lost or stolen in each breach.

- The three main reasons for a data breach were lost or stolen computing devices, employee mistakes, and third-party snafus.

- Fifty-two percent of organizations discovered the data breach as a result of an audit or assessment, the rest from employees detecting the breach.

- Fifty-four percent of organizations have little or no confidence that their organization can detect all patient data loss or theft.

- Ninety-one percent of hospitals surveyed are using cloud-based services, yet 47 percent lack confidence in the ability to keep data secure in the cloud.

Despite recent attacks on medical devices, 69 percent of respondents say their organization's IT security and/or data protection activities do not include the security of FDA-approved medical devices.

"Healthcare organizations seem to face an uphill battle in their efforts to stop and reduce the loss or theft of protected health information (PHI) or patient information."

Ponemon Institute.
Third Annual Benchmark Study on Patient Privacy
& Data Security.

Trust No One

The headlines might be filled with reports of cyberspying by individuals in China and Russia, but when it comes to patient data, your biggest worry should be your employees. The Ponemon report found that "insider negligence continues to be at the root of the data breach." Nearly half (46 percent) of security breaches were attributed to lost or stolen computing devices, often due to employee, well, negligence. However, criminal attacks have also increased and are now responsible for a third of security breaches, up from 20 percent in 2010.

Part of the problem may be that most healthcare systems (81 percent of those in the Ponemon survey) allow employees and medical staff to use their own mobile devices to connect to system networks or email, despite serious concerns about their security. It's called bring your own device (BYOD).

"Health care organizations are ... implementing BYOD in which the security is absolutely and totally inadequate," said Dr. Braithwaite. "That makes my hair stand on end." The devices "get stolen right and left," he said.

Indeed, there are reports of people having their smartphones or tablets snatched from their hands while using them. A 2013 article in *Time* magazine reported that about half of all robberies in San Francisco now involve a mobile phone, while a Harris Poll found that nearly 10 percent of cellular users said their phones had been stolen.[49] The U.S. Department of Health and Human Services (HHS) attributes nearly 40 percent of large HIPAA rule violations to lost or stolen devices.[50]

"Health care faces unique BYOD challenges because of privacy and security regulations," said David Ting, founder and chief technology officer of Imprivata, in an interview with *HIT Consultant Media*. His company markets HIPAA-compliant text messaging systems to healthcare organizations. Chief information officers, he said, need to understand the risks and approach the problem with the right mind-set.[51]

One risk is that employees who use their own devices that are connected to a healthcare system's IT infrastructure increase the risk of malware to the entire system. Indeed, a report from Boston-based cybercrime analyst Trusteer predicted that more than 5 percent of all iOS and Android smartphones were infected with malware in 2012. That's a statistic we should take to heart given that an estimated 80 percent of physicians use one or the other device.[52]

Sinko calls personal devices and personal uses of institutional devices the "STDs of malware" because it introduces weak points into the IT ecosystem. "Every weekend, I take my laptop home and go into the *Sports Illustrated* website," he explains. "If there is malware in that website, then anyone who visits the site can have the tiny bits of software installed on their computer." All Cleveland Clinic devices have malware protection installed; few personal devices do. "It's scary to think about how much malware is out there that institutions don't know about," he said.

"Any time you bring a new device into your system, think of it as already compromised," Ting said in the interview. "It's a device you have no control over that has been used as a personal device rather than a professional instrument. It could have malware on it. It may have none, but the weakest link is where your breach is going to be, so it's imperative to begin your BYOD plan with that assumption."[51]

The 2012 HIMSS Mobile Health Survey found that nearly all of the 180 organizations surveyed either had a mobile technology plan in place or were developing one. About three-quarters of those with policies addressed the issue of BYOD.[6]

If your organization/practice has decided to allow employees to use their own devices for patient care, you need to consider the following in developing any policy:

- What are the risks of bringing an "unclean" machine into the organization?

- How will we support these devices?

- What system and infrastructure requirements are needed? For instance, will the additional devices overburden our Wi-Fi system?

- How can we guarantee and enforce endpoint security? That includes the ability to authenticate the user.

Enterprise application software developer SAP uses its own Afaria mobile device management program to manage and secure its BYOD program, which involves more than 40,000 mobile devices across the globe. Regardless of which program you use, the company recommends considering the following:

- What is your mobile strategy? How do you anticipate employees using mobile devices?

- Will access to company data vary based on whether the company or the employee owns the device?

- Which employees can access enterprise data?

- Is the enterprise or patient data stored locally on the device?

- What devices will you support?

- How can you meet privacy and data protection laws and regulations with a BYOD strategy?

- Should employees sign contracts and, if so, what should the contracts contain?

- Will employees be able to access unapproved applications from their company-owned devices? What about personal devices during work hours?

- How will you handle termination or when someone leaves the company?

- Who pays for the devices and repairs, as well as accessories like chargers?

- Who pays for the voice and data plan, including roaming charges during travel and apps?

- How should you handle "jailbroken" or "rooted" devices, which remove all software/firmware restrictions on the device.

- How should devices be secured? What happens if an employee reports a lost device? Should the entire device be remotely wiped or only company data?

- How do you ensure compliance with the BYOD policy, and what are the repercussions for those who do not comply?

- Will you allow backup to the cloud and use of cloud-based file-sharing programs?

- Should employees be able to use cameras, Bluetooth, or other applications and services for work-related uses?

- Can you enforce passwords on the whole device?

Ting's company also offers tools to help maintain the integrity of endpoint security, such as its OneSign Anywhere, which provides strong authentication and single sign-on capabilities (automated username and password entry for authenticated users) for devices at remote locations or within an organization. This enables organizations to control the exposure of any internal applications. Other companies sell similar products.

Rick Kam, president of the security firm ID Experts, suggested other steps you should take in a 2011 *FierceMobileHealthcare* article:[52]

- Don't allow wireless devices to store patient data and, if you do, make sure it's encrypted.

- Make sure all mobile devices are password protected and that the screen locks down after a minute or two of inactivity.

- Turn on the "remote wipe" feature of all wireless devices.

- Use the newest version of Wi-Fi–protected access protocols.

- Change your system's default service set identifier (SSID) and administration passwords regularly.

- Don't transmit your wireless router's SSID.

- Require mobile devices to identify themselves via their media access control (MAC) address before logging into the network.

- Implement a wireless intrusion prevention system.

Figure 2-1. Five Steps to Manage Your Mobile Device

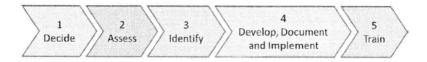

1. Decide whether mobile devices will be used to access, receive, transmit, or store patients' health information or used as part of your organization's internal networks or systems (e.g., your electronic health system).

2. Consider how mobile devices affect the risks (threats and vulnerabilities) to the health information your organization holds.

3. Identify your organization's mobile device risk management strategy, including privacy and security safeguards.

4. Develop, document, and implement the organization's mobile policies and procedures to safeguard health information.

5. Conduct mobile device privacy and security awareness and training for providers and professionals.

In the Cloud

While providers may protect mobile devices with the ability to wipe data remotely if the device is stolen or lost, they don't have that same ability with data stored in the cloud. While the storage itself might be secure, providers need to consider the security of data transmitted between the cloud and the device. They should also ask what happens if the cloud gets hacked. It's not a hypothetical question; in the past year, hackers have hit several high-profile companies, including *The New York Times*, Zappos, Google, *The Wall Street Journal*, and General Motors.

Many providers aren't aware of the risks. A Chicago hospital system used an unsecured Dropbox site for new residents managing patient care through iPads. The Dropbox had a single user name and password for all users. Even more stunning? The user name and password were published in a manual online. The medical center only changed the system after a *Washington Post* reporter called about it.[41]

Although the medical center told the *Post* that the system was only meant to share educational material, a security expert explained in the article that this approach still exposed the medical center to "social engineering" attacks, in which hackers plant documents with malicious code. Once opened, the code could infect the iPads, providing access to hospital networks.

The Foundation of Healthcare Privacy: HIPAA

The issue of patient privacy didn't become front and center until 1996, when Congress passed the Health Insurance Portability and Accountability Act, known as HIPAA.

In a nutshell, the rule provides federal protections for protected health information (PHI) held by "covered entities," i.e., doctors, hospitals, nursing homes, dentists, physical therapists, chiropractors, payers, clearinghouses—anyone who treats a patient and anywhere a patient receives any type of medical care. It also provides an array of patient rights regarding that information. For instance, patients can approve the disclosure of their information to whomever they wish. Disclosing anything without that permission, however, subjects the "covered entity" to hefty fines.

Those fines got a lot heftier and the regulations much broader with the release in 2013 of the largest overhaul of HIPAA since its implementation. A major part of that overhaul? Clarifying previous assumptions that, yes, HIPAA does apply to all mobile applications and mobile uses of health information technology. The new rules also apply HIPAA regulations to the business associates and contractors of covered entities. This includes cloud providers, health information exchanges, and EHR vendors that host applications, to name just a few.

The new regulations should be a wake-up call for any healthcare entity, says Sirois, particularly those sharing data wirelessly. Below, she highlights the ramifications of the new law:

- **HIPAA coverage expanded.** HIPAA now applies not only to covered entities, but to *their* vendors and business associates. So if a company sells a mobile EHR app to a hospital and has access to personal health information as part of the app support, and the security of that app is compromised and puts patient data at risk, the vendor is liable for the same fines as the covered entity.

- **HIPAA penalties are going to hurt.** Previously, civil monetary penalties were limited to a maximum of $100 per violation with a $25,000 annual cap for similar violations. Now, penalties range from $100 to $50,000 each (Table 1), with a $1.5 million annual cap for multiple violations of identical provisions and criminal penalties of up to 10 years imprisonment.

- **Ignorance of the law is no excuse.** Willful neglect, defined as "conscious, intentional failure or reckless indifference to the obligation to comply with the administrative simplification provision violated," or, in other words, "you knew-your-system-wasn't-secure-but-hoped-we-wouldn't-notice," is at the top of the scale of penalties. HHS can impose penalties at even the mere possibility of a violation due to willful neglect. Even an honest mistake such as emailing patient health data to the wrong patient can be considered willful neglect if the mistake was not handled through the appropriate corporate compliance channels. So "neglecting" to protect mHealth devices or educate users on privacy and security requirements is a tremendous risk, to say the least!

> *"This final Omnibus Rule marks the most sweeping change to the HIPAA privacy and security rules since they were first implemented. These changes not only greatly enhance a patient's privacy rights and protections, but also strengthen the ability of my office to vigorously enforce the HIPAA privacy and security protections, regardless of whether the information is being held by a health plan, a health care provider, or one of their business associates."*

Leon Rodriguez
HHS Office for Civil Rights Director.

Table 2-1. Tiers of Civil Monetary Penalties (CMP) Related to Level of Culpability

Violation Category	Each Violation	Total CMP for Violations of an Identical Provision in a Calendar Year
Unknowing	$100-$50,000	$1,500,000
Reasonable cause	$1,000-$50,000	$1,500,000
Willful neglect, corrected	$10,000-$50,000	$1,500,000
Willful neglect, not corrected	At least $50,000	$1,500,000

Implementing the New HIPAA Rules

Dr. Braithwaite helped draft the original HIPAA law in 1994, when the Internet was still novel and cellphones were the size of bricks. Even then, he said, the security law was designed to adapt to technological changes. "It's critical that people understand that the security rule requires a very simple underlying process: you have to identify and assess any risks or threats to the electronic information, not just to its confidentiality, but to its availability and integrity as well."

That means assessing the risks and figuring out how to manage those risks by implementing *appropriate and reasonable administrative, physical, and technical safeguards.* "That term 'appropriate and reasonable' was used 75 times in the security rule alone," Dr. Braithwaite noted. It allows institutions to consider their size, complexity, technical infrastructure, hardware and software capabilities, cost, and probability and size of potential risks. "Then you educate and train your people, you document and monitor what's going on, and you repeat this cycle over and over again forever."

"HIPAA didn't say you must encrypt this or you must do this or you must do that," he said. "It says, 'Figure out what the threats are, figure out what the risks are, and do something to prevent those risks from causing you problems.'"

Table 2-2. When Does HIPAA Apply?

Scenario	HIPAA Applies
Mobile app clinicians and others use to access electronic health record	Yes
Mobile app patients use to access their EHR	Maybe
Reminder texts sent to patients about their appointments	Yes
Medical information sent by patients that physicians access	No
Insurance company's mobile app that collects patient claims data/information	Yes
Application that provides statistics on influenza immunization in a specific geographic area	No
Application that allows a nurse to add information about patients who received their flu shots	Yes
Data beamed to medical device company from defibrillator implanted in patient's chest	Maybe

Moving Beyond HIPAA: The Security of Medical Devices

"Privacy regulations are not enough when you can literally alter data used by clinicians to make life or death decisions. If you compromise health care and shake people's confidence in a doctor's ability to safely treat patients, then follow that with a biological attack, even a small one, a terrorist would have one seriously successful attack."

John Gomez, CEO,
Sensato
Interview with HISTalk, September 19, 2011

Although much of the focus on mHealth "security" revolves around HIPAA, those rules are about privacy—they don't set security rules. And when it comes to the healthcare system, security is about more than just stealing identities or patient records; it's about life and death. Healthcare providers need to realize that if a device can send data *out,* then someone can send data *in*, potentially compromising not only integrity of the information the healthcare provider receives, but patient safety.

Consider a diabetes patient with an implantable insulin pump that is controlled by a remote device over the airways and sends information via the Internet to the patient's doctor. What if someone hacked into it and changed the settings, sending a bolus of insulin into the patient's veins that could injure or even kill him? It's not science fiction. One of Gomez's colleagues, who has an implantable insulin pump, demonstrated this possibility using his laptop and Web browser over a public wireless network.

During a presentation at the Breakpoint 2012 Security Conference in Australia, a premier meeting for security information technology experts, one presenter showed how someone with a laptop standing 50 feet away could deliver a fatal, 830-volt shock to a pacemaker patient.[53] At the DEF CON 19 Conference in Las Vegas in 2011, 1,100 hackers attended a session on "Hacking Healthcare" and learned to attack MRI and CT scanners. This could allow them to manipulate the image quality and scan time; reverse engineer the device or infect it with malware or viruses; or attach a device to the MRI machine and control it remotely.

The Ponemon survey found that 69 percent of organizations surveyed did not secure their medical devices, possibly because they think it's the vendor's responsibility. The reality is that if a privacy breach occurs, both are responsible—and both face steep HIPAA fines.[46]

And a 2012 report from the General Accounting Office found the threat of malicious interventions to implantable wireless devices so significant that it recommended the U.S. Food and Drug Administration (FDA) develop a plan to address them. It was somewhat frightening to read in the report that the FDA had *never even considered* security risks from *intentional* threats until it saw an early draft of the report.[54]

Catch 22: A True Story

Don Sinko tells a story about coming into work one Monday to find that someone had pried off the laptop part of a medical device and stolen it. The laptop contained sensitive medical information. The FDA-approved device was not encrypted, "and we couldn't encrypt it because then we would override the FDA approval," he said. It's a Catch-22 conundrum that he is pursuing with the Office of Civil Rights, which oversees HIPAA.

Even if the FDA starts requiring encryption on all medical devices, that ruling won't apply to devices already in use—and healthcare entities are unlikely to commit the enormous capital that would be required to replace them.

Sinko brings up another concern with medical devices: liability. "If the doctor implants a defibrillator that sends data to her computer 24 hours a day, and that defibrillator is hacked, who is responsible? The doctor or the company that made the device?"

"Chances are, if it is in a hospital and taking care of a patient, it has an IP address and can be hacked."

John Gomez, CEO,
Sensato

"Security," says Gomez bluntly, "is about securing people and ensuring that when they're moving around (with a medical device) someone can't hack into their device and literally try to assault or kill them."

Who Owns Medical Device Data?

A 2012 article in *The Wall Street Journal* raised an interesting question: Does a patient have a right to data sent from an implantable device to a doctor or device company, and can the device company sell that data to health systems and insurers to use in algorithms to predict disease?

In the article, the doctors interviewed said they thought that patients should have access to that data; but the device makers did not. The manufacturers said it would be too cumbersome to provide such data, that it would require FDA approval (which it most likely would not), and that under federal regulations (presumably HIPAA), only doctors and other medical professionals have access to that data. What's not clear, the article concluded, is whether HIPAA regulations *do* apply to devices.

"Is the device itself a depository for medical records?" asked Paul C. Zei, M.D., a cardiologist at Stanford University Medical Center, in the article. His patient wanted the same access to his cardiac-device data as the doctor. "Or is it part of the patient, and an extension of vital signs that we download into a medical chart?"[55]

Just one more thing to figure out in the Brave New World of mHealth.

Don't Forget Patient Generated Data and Patient Apps

Much of the discussion about privacy and security focuses on the role of the provider in keeping data safe. But how do you protect patient-provided health information, such as that shared through a personal cellphone, tablet, or computer, or directly entered into a personal health record? What about data entered into exercise or nutrition apps on a smartphone?

Currently, the Robert Wood Johnson Foundation notes, there are no clear legal standards on this. It recommends that providers involve themselves in patient information security in both provider-led and non-provider-led initiatives. Foundation experts also recommend information encryption for personal health information sent via text message, educating patients about the risks of unencrypted text messages, and instructing patients to limit the extent of personal health information they send over unencrypted channels.[56]

Dr. Braithwaite envisions a scenario in which someone enters information into a diabetes app and the data is sold to an employer, bank, or mortgage company, which can then discriminate against that individual. "We are using health information about people to discriminate against them in ways that ought to be preventable in the same way as you shouldn't be using a person's age or their gender or their skin color to discriminate against them," he said. The Omnibus Rule specifically addressed the security and privacy of genetic information utilization and nondiscrimination, but there's a lot of other information about us that could be used to discriminate against us in numerous ways.

Breaking Down Barriers

So, what's going on? Why can't healthcare organizations get their privacy/security houses in order? The answers aren't surprising: a shortage of technology, funding, and expertise. And, as we have seen, the continuously and rapidly shifting environment as technology evolves and hackers and thieves become more creative and determined to infiltrate it.

Yet, there is no dearth of consultants eager to help companies improve their mobile security. In fact, research firm IDC says global spending on mobile security is on track to balloon to $1.9 billion by 2015, up from $407 million in 2010.[57]

Enter government regulation and consumer demand.

In February 2013, the Federal Trade Commission (FTC) found that more than half of all app users (57 percent) have either uninstalled an app over concerns about sharing their personal information or chose not to install such an app in the first place. In addition, less than one-third of Americans feel they are in control of their personal information on their mobile devices.

In response, the FTC issued the following recommendations for platform developers:

- Provide just-in-time disclosures to consumers and obtain their affirmative express consent before allowing apps to access sensitive content like geolocation.

- Provide just-in-time disclosures and obtain affirmative express consent for other content that consumers would find sensitive in many contexts, such as contacts, photos, calendar entries, or the recording of audio or video content.

- Develop a one-stop "dashboard" approach to allow consumers to review the types of content accessed by the apps they have downloaded.

- Develop icons to depict the transmission of user data.

- Promote app developer best practices: require developers to make privacy disclosures, reasonably enforce these requirements, and educate app developers.

- Provide consumers with clear disclosures about the extent to which platforms review apps prior to making them available for download in the app stores and conduct compliance checks after the apps have been placed in the app stores.

- Offer a do not track (DNT) mechanism for smartphone users that would allow consumers to choose to prevent tracking by ad networks or other third parties as they navigate among apps on their phones.

In addition, the FTC cited specific recommendations for application developers:

- Have a privacy policy and make sure it is easily accessible through the app stores.

- Provide just-in-time disclosures and obtain affirmative express consent before collecting and sharing sensitive information (if the platforms have not already disclosed the information and obtained consent).

- Improve coordination and communication with ad networks and other third parties that provide services for apps, such as analytics companies, so the app developers can better understand the software they are using and, in turn, provide accurate disclosures to consumers.

- Participate in self-regulatory programs, trade associations, and industry organizations, which can provide guidance on how to make uniform, short-form privacy disclosures.

In a Perspective piece in the February 27, 2013, *New England Journal of Medicine,* Julie K. Taitsman, M.D., J.D., and colleagues from HHS's Office of the Inspector General provided several "best practices" that healthcare organizations should follow to protect EHRs and other patient information:[8]

- Implement strong security measures such as password protection, firewalls, and antivirus software.

- Require that staff sign in and out of various devices as they go from room to room, and that all programs be equipped with automatic logouts.

- Develop audit trails.

- Vet all personnel with access to patient information, including background checks.

- Train all staff on "appropriate information sharing," and when they leave the organization, deactivate all access to records.

- Make sure all security provisions follow staff home.

Healthcare systems and providers will have to tighten security if they want to partake of the millions available in federal health information technology money. Meaningful Use Stage 2, which sets requirements for how EHRs should be used in order to receive federal incentive monies, requires that providers and hospitals conduct risk analyses for data security on mobile devices, that patients have secure access to their medical information, and that data stored in EHRs on mobile devices or applications, or any personal health information on such devices, be encrypted.[58]

The healthcare industry, says Dr. Braithwaite, should follow in the footsteps of the banking industry, with formal processes for identity proofing and with multifactor authentication and monitoring of transactions. Third-party companies like Kintera, Equifax, and AT&T now offer services to certify third parties with secure proofing and authentication.

The two main reasons healthcare organizations don't take advantage of such services, Dr. Braithwaite said, is that they erroneously think it will be too expensive and that patients will balk at any lengthy requirement to access their own medical records. That won't happen, he said.

When he worked at Equifax, he helped design an EHR website where patients could retrieve their medical records and communicate with their doctors. The site used strong, knowledge-based identity proofing and multifactorial authentication, he said, "and the patients loved it. They said, 'Finally, you're paying attention to the security of my sensitive information, so I trust you now and I will go use it.'"

At the Cleveland Clinic, our team takes these issues very seriously. We use two-factor authentication for remote access and, although we're moving toward BYOD, we are doing so in a very thoughtful, deliberate manner, asking the questions highlighted throughout this chapter. Devices will have to be configured to our standards and be remotely wipeable if they are lost or stolen.

Smaller hospitals, however, don't have our depth of resources. That's why Sinko says some of the BYOD security issues need to be addressed by the device makers themselves. There was a reason Blackberry was the phone of choice in the corporate world for years, he said, because the company understood the security risks and designed the phone to protect the data. The Android and iOS operating systems don't have the enterprise level security that Blackberry built. Instead, companies building devices that use these operating systems appear to have abandoned enterprise security for the consumer-driven bells and whistles of newer devices.

Will You Certify Your App?

Happtique, a mobile health applications store and evaluation service, released its own standards for testing and certifying mobile health apps in February 2013.

The standards are designed to enable healthcare organizations to assess the content, operability, privacy, and security of mobile health apps. A panel composed of recognized leaders in mHealth, healthcare technology, healthcare certification and accreditation programs, and patient advocacy, along with input from healthcare and information technology organizations and representatives of key federal agencies (FDA, Federal Communications Commission, FTC, and the Office of the National Coordinator for Health Information Technology), developed the standards. The London-based testing and certification company Intertek will evaluate the apps and, once they pass the technical tests, send them on to medical organizations to assess the

Will You Certify Your App?

accuracy of any content.[59]

From the Office of the National Coordinator for Health Information Technology

The federal Office of the National Coordinator for Health Information Technology, which is the principal federal entity charged with coordination of nationwide efforts to implement and use the most advanced health information technology and the electronic exchange of health information, recommends the following for managing mobile devices in healthcare environments:[60]

- ✓ Decide whether mobile devices will be used to access, receive, transmit, or store patients' health information or be used as part of your organization's internal network or systems, such as an EHR system. Understand the risks to your organization before you decide to allow the use of mobile devices.

- ✓ Consider the risks when using mobile devices to transmit the health information your organization holds. Conduct a risk analysis to identify threats and vulnerabilities. If you are a solo provider, you may conduct the risk analysis yourself. If you work for a large provider, the organization may conduct it.

- ✓ Identify a mobile device risk management strategy, including privacy and security safeguards. A risk management strategy will help your organization develop and implement mobile device safeguards to reduce risks identified in the risk analysis, including evaluation and regular maintenance of the mobile device safeguards you put in place.

- ✓ Conduct mobile device privacy and security awareness and ongoing training for providers, employees, and professionals.

✓ Develop, document, and implement your organization's mobile device policies and procedures to safeguard health information. Some topics to consider when developing mobile device policies and procedures are:

- o Mobile device management
- o Using your own device
- o Restrictions on mobile device use
- o Security or configuration settings for mobile devices.

Texting to Patients

An increasing number of healthcare organizations are using text messages to reach patients with health-related information. They had better be careful not to overstep. Researchers from Washington state evaluated two text messages developed for a campaign to send reminders to parents whose child required a second flu shot.[61] The researchers' analysis of various texts and the potential HIPAA implications are shown in Figure 2-2.

Figure 2-2. Flu Shot Reminders Texts

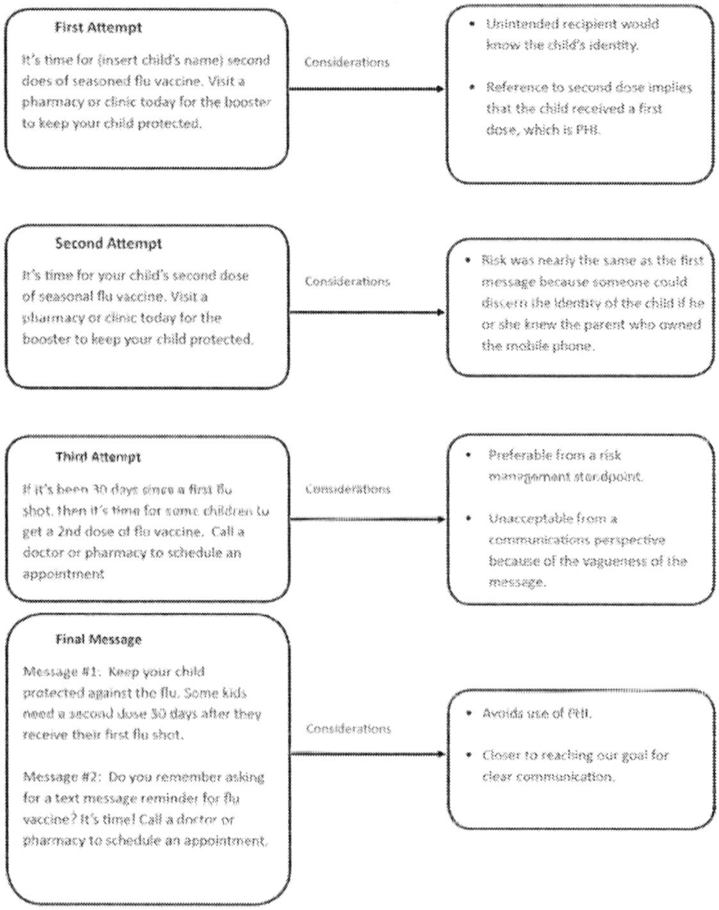

First Attempt

It's time for (insert child's name) second dose of seasoned flu vaccine. Visit a pharmacy or clinic today for the booster to keep your child protected.

Considerations →

- Unintended recipient would know the child's identity.
- Reference to second dose implies that the child received a first dose, which is PHI.

Second Attempt

It's time for your child's second dose of seasonal flu vaccine. Visit a pharmacy or clinic today for the booster to keep your child protected.

Considerations →

- Risk was nearly the same as the first message because someone could discern the identity of the child if he or she knew the parent who owned the mobile phone.

Third Attempt

If it's been 30 days since a first flu shot, then it's time for some children to get a 2nd dose of flu vaccine. Call a doctor or pharmacy to schedule an appointment

Considerations →

- Preferable from a risk management standpoint.
- Unacceptable from a communications perspective because of the vagueness of the message.

Final Message

Message #1: Keep your child protected against the flu. Some kids need a second dose 30 days after they receive their first flu shot.

Message #2: Do you remember asking for a text message reminder for flu vaccine? It's time! Call a doctor or pharmacy to schedule an appointment.

Considerations →

- Avoids use of PHI.
- Closer to reaching our goal for clear communication.

Note. PHI = protected health information.

Source: Karasz HN, Eiden A, Bogan S. Text Messaging to Communicate With Public Health Audiences: How the HIPAA Security Rule Affects Practice. *Am J Public Health.* 2013: e1-e7.

Chapter 2: Key Takeaways

✓ Despite the promise of mHealth, it faces significant barriers in the areas of privacy and security.

✓ Barriers are evident not only in terms of the electronic and personal health records, but also with the plethora of medical devices that are connected to the Internet and/or transmit data wirelessly.

✓ Protecting privacy does not translate into security.

✓ Having security measures in place does not translate to privacy.

✓ The healthcare system lags behind nearly every other industry in terms of information security.

✓ Spending on mobile security continues to rise exponentially, a trend that is unlikely to plateau in the next five years.

✓ Employees who use their own devices to access patient information put the entire institution's information technology system at risk.

✓ Federal regulation of security and privacy issues around mHealth is growing.

✓ New HIPAA rules expand the role of the privacy law in mHealth.

Chapter 3. mHealth in the Clinical Setting: the Need for Disruptive Change

"Consumers are ready to adopt mobile health faster than the health care industry is ready to adapt."

PwC
Emerging mHealth: Paths for Growth. June 2012

Ryan Sysko's sister, an endocrinologist at the Joslin Diabetes Center in Boston, was frustrated and disillusioned with the current state of diabetes care. Trying to teach her patients to manage their diabetes, she told her brother, was like trying to teach them a foreign language in four, 15-minute sessions. Instead of managing her patients proactively based on real-time information on their status, everything she did was retrospective, based on their glucose readings over the past three months. And no matter how much she tried to educate her patients, a few months later they'd forgotten everything. And no wonder. "These are people with multiple jobs, families to deal with ... trying to (manage their diabetes) is very burdensome," she told him.

She noticed one thing. Even though she practiced in a predominately low-income area, every patient had a cellphone. While they might leave their homes without their glucose meters, they never left home without their cellphones. How, she and Ryan wondered, could they harness the potential of the device to improve diabetes care?

Thus was born DiabetesManager, the first app from Baltimore-based WellDoc. Today, WellDoc is a leading provider of diabetes-management mHealth applications and software.

The company's cornerstone product provides real-time, longitudinal feedback to patients based on their glucose levels and other clinical metrics. It also sends that information to their clinicians, along with evidence-based recommendations to improve glucose management.

To prove their app worked and get provider and payer buy-in, the company turned to the gold standard in medical research: a controlled, randomized clinical trial. Its Mobile Diabetes Intervention Study assigned 163 patients from 26 primary care practices to one of three stepped treatment groups—the mobile and Web-based patient coaching system involving patients and providers; a provider-only portal; a provider-only portal linked to standards of care and evidence-based guidelines; or to usual care (the control group). After one year, those in the mobile- and Web-based app group demonstrated clinically significant improvement in their diabetes management, with a nearly 2 percent decline in their hemoglobin A1C levels compared to a 0.7 percent decline in the usual care group.[62]

Further proof of DiabetesManager's effectiveness came from a demonstration program sponsored by the District of Columbia Department of Health and conducted by George Washington University Medical Center. The 32 Medicaid patients enrolled in the pilot reduced their emergency department (ED) visits and hospital stays by 58 percent compared to the 12 months before the program.[63] The Food and Drug Administration (FDA) gave the company 510(K) clearance to market the device, basically approving it as a medical device. It is available for most mobile phones, is prescribed by physicians, and is reimbursed by many health plans.

With its app, WellDoc has the potential to improve diabetes outcomes on a large scale, something that is desperately needed, given that 25.8 million people, or 8.3 percent of the U.S. population, have diabetes.[64] Globally, an estimated 6.4 percent of adults, about 285 million, had diabetes in 2010, a prevalence expected to increase to 7.7 percent (439 million adults) by 2030, with the majority of the increase occurring in developing countries.[65]

WellDoc's app demonstrates the power of mHealth to address complex, frustrating issues within the healthcare system. Those issues, however, lie not just in the clinical realm, but in the quality and financial realms, as well. They lie in changing the way medicine is practiced, breaking down provider siloes, and encouraging patient engagement and provider collaboration.

While mHealth is not the sole answer, it is a major piece of the puzzle as we work to improve quality and reduce the cost of health care. In other words, adding mHealth to current healthcare delivery models provides a powerful new ally in our quest to better manage health.

Time for Change

How do you change a 100-year-old business model? That's the question we have to ask—and the challenge we have to address—as we roll out mHealth to healthcare providers. Engaging physicians, nurses, therapists, and large healthcare systems in mHealth requires changing the paradigm they are accustomed to, a paradigm that often puts the provider first and the patient second. It requires a shift in the reimbursement structure. And it requires a shift in our understanding of what it means to practice medicine.

In short, it requires what is often called a "disruptive innovation." We didn't coin the term. That came from Harvard Business School professor Clayton M. Christensen, who, in a 2000 *Harvard Business Review* article, described the U.S. healthcare system as "the most entrenched change-averse industry" in the country.[66]

However, he wrote, given that the "transformational force" of disruptive innovation brought affordability and accessibility to other industries, it must inevitably come to health care. He highlighted three enablers of disruptive innovation: a simplifying technology, business model innovation, and a disruptive value network.[67] mHealth technology can meet all of those criteria if designed and implemented appropriately.

The good news is that provider resistance is weakening. Medical school students and residents, who grew up with smartphones, tablets, and wireless everything, are already demanding—and expecting—that such tools be integrated into their education and clinical management. We find this in the courses we teach in our medical school. At the Cleveland Clinic Lerner College of Medicine, the entire curriculum is available through a custom-learning portal. The number one frustration for students is when content from seminars is not posted and accessible online.

This generation expects 24/7 access to everything—including their patients. We've seen young physicians completely flummoxed when our computer system goes down. They don't know what to do because they've never taken care of patients without a computer (something that is also problematic).

This momentum is, by necessity, spilling over into the older generation, which is still in transition from thinking "*What* is this computer?" to "*Where* is my computer?" Yet doctors and nurses are no different from anyone else when it comes to their uptake of smartphones and other mobile devices. More than half of doctors surveyed by the University of Kansas School of Medicine-Wichita in 2012 reported that they send and receive work-related texts even when they're not on call,[68] while a 2012 survey from Spyglass Consulting Group found that 69 percent of surveyed hospital nurses said they use their smartphones for personal and clinical communications while on the job.[69]

Meanwhile, the 2012 HIMSS Mobile Technology Survey found that the use of mobile technology to collect data at the bedside rose to 45 percent in 2012, a 30 percent jump over the previous year, while the use of such technology to monitor medical device data is now 34 percent.[6]

The increased use of communication such as texts, email, and even interactions in social media groups with patients has caught the attention of the American College of Physicians and the Federation of State Medical Boards, which issued a policy statement on online medical professionalism between patients and physicians.[70]

Among the recommendations:

- Develop guidelines that spell out what issues are appropriate for electronic communication, and use this form of communication only with patients who follow up in person.

- Maintain patient confidentiality. "The sharing of patient information must always be held to a higher level of security than standard residential Internet connections." That means encrypted or virtual proxy network connections for hospital-based systems, institutional policies on home-based access to and use of such information, and remote monitoring of cellphones and tablets to "wipe" any data if they are lost or stolen.

- Stay off public, unsecured wireless and cellular networks for patient and/or physician communication.

- Keep in mind that written communication, missing the nonverbal aspects of face-to-face communication, is prone to misunderstanding.

- Make sure you know *why* you are communicating electronically rather than verbally.

The New Drugstore Shopping List: Shampoo, Mascara, and Sinusitis Diagnosis

Large drugstore chains like Walgreens and CVS have been active in the "mini-clinic" movement for years, running walk-in clinics in their stores staffed by nurse practitioners and pharmacists who diagnose and treat most minor conditions like sinusitis and bronchitis. Now, however, they're taking those clinics virtual. In 2012, Rite Aid announced it would open 58 stores in Baltimore, Boston, Philadelphia, and Pittsburgh with in-store clinics that provide virtual doctor visits via Web camera.

Patients pay $45 for a 10-minute virtual consultation. Although patients currently self-pay, the chain expects insurers will eventually cover the visits.

Electronic Health Records: What Happened?

There is, however, one big challenge we face to successful implementation: the current state of the electronic health record (EHR).

Although it might sound like an oxymoron, we think that underdeveloped countries with relatively nonexistent healthcare systems are in a far better situation when it comes to implementing mHealth than industrialized countries like the United States. That's because they don't have to "shoehorn" new technology and a new way of doing business into an existing behemoth of a system that embraces systemic change with all the enthusiasm of someone facing their first colonoscopy.

Instead, they can build the system on the backbone of mHealth technology, which, as you'll see in Chapter 6, is exactly what countries like Nigeria, Tanzania, and Ghana are doing. In the United States and other Western countries, however, we have to first overcome our innate resistance to certain forms of technology. We're not talking about "traditional" technology like imaging, laboratory tests, or robotic surgery, which clinicians are often quick to adopt. No, we are talking about the challenges of the EHR.

The rollout of the EHR over the past 20 years has been a complex undertaking with mixed results. An analysis by the RAND Corporation released in early 2013 found that the productivity and quality benefits RAND predicted in a 2005 analysis have not materialized.[71] A 2012 study published in the *Journal of the American Medical Association* reported similar findings: differences in productivity in hospitals with high penetration of EHRs was related not to the digital information, but to the fact that they employ more nurses.[72]

The issues with EHRs are important for two reasons: their impact on clinician trust of other digital technologies designed to improve quality and reduce costs; and the need to integrate mHealth technologies with existing EHRs, which is a nonnegotiable part of the mHealth rollout.

The EHR and mHealth apps and devices should work synergistically, with the apps and devices feeding data into the EHR, and patients and providers accessing and updating the EHR remotely with mHealth apps and devices.

That's exactly what we're doing at the Cleveland Clinic. We created an app called Well-Q that we give to patients a few days before a scheduled visit with their primary care physician. They use the app to complete a comprehensive wellness assessment on an iPad that takes just a few minutes. Nothing too exciting about that. But the data from that app feeds directly into the patient's EHR and creates "flags" for the physician.

For instance, if the patient is a smoker, the physician will have smoking cessation orders as well as patient education teed up for the office visit. By integrating patient entered data with data that is within the EHR, we can deploy more accurate disease screen algorithms. So, while the app assesses the patient for smoking behaviors and symptoms, the clinician has a better prediction for their risk of chronic obstructive pulmonary disorder (COPD).

We used intelligent design to "learn" from the patient's answers and adjust the screening questions and responses accordingly. So, for instance, if the patient's responses to the first two questions on the depression screen are negative, they don't have to complete the rest of the screen. Other areas we assess include nutrition, sleep and exercise. Not only do physicians receive prompts based on the data, but patients are also provided education and materials based on their responses. For instance, if their responses suggest a poor diet, they receive nutritional information.

When we tested the app over 90 days at one of our primary care centers, we found overwhelming patient support, even from patients you'd think would shy away from technology, like the 70-year-old Amish couple who were one of our first testers. Our physicians liked it too. They told us it enabled them to have conversations with patients that they wouldn't have had otherwise.

We need these kinds of apps—and their ability to seamlessly integrate into the EHR and enhance, not disrupt, the work flow—if we are to realize the promise of population-based health care that so much of healthcare reform is built on.

Our goal, and it should be the goal of every healthcare organization out there, is to get the right information to the right person in the right format at the right time with the right device. In our minds, this should be the Golden Rule of mHealth.

Meaningful Use and mHealth

The Health Information Technology for Economic and Clinical Health (HITECH) Act of 2009 provides incentives and, beginning in 2015, disincentives, to encourage the use of EHRs. The technology must be used for more than just record keeping, however. HHS has been releasing regulations spelling out the requirements for financial bonuses under HITECH, requirements designed to ensure "Meaningful Use" of EHRs.

That means using EHRSs to provide complete and accurate information; better access to information that can be shared across healthcare settings, ideally improving coordinate of care; and patient empowerment, encouraging patients to take a more active role in their health and the health of their families.

Several stages of meaningful use requirements will be released; the first two are already in effect. "Meaningful use is the engine that converts policy into practice," said C. Martin Harris, M.D., chief information offices at the Cleveland Clinic. Unfortunately, he said, there's been too much focus on Stages 1 and 2—adoption and interoperability. The true promise of EHRs and mHealth will come with later stages, he said. He also warns that "it's not about the tools, but about how to restructure the healthcare delivery system."

What Happened with EHRs?

There are many reasons for the lost opportunities we've seen with the EHR rollout that hold valuable lessons as we roll out mHealth.

They include:

- Information technology (IT) systems in many physician offices, hospitals, pharmacies, health plans, and other healthcare entities are not interoperable and rarely "talk to each other." This limits one goal of EHRs (and mHealth): to improve coordination of care between healthcare settings and providers. This is already a problem in the mHealth realm. A PwC survey found that just half of the 433 doctors interviewed said the mHealth applications and services they used worked with their organization's information technology. Far fewer said the applications they used were well integrated with the IT systems of local hospitals and clinics, national healthcare systems, or systems that colleagues accessed in other organizations.[30]

In addition, only about a quarter of the 130 IT professionals polled for the 2012 HIMSS Mobile Technology Survey said the data their physicians captured with mobile devices was fully integrated with patients' EHRs, even though 45 percent used mobile devices to collect data at the patient's bedside.[6]

- The slow adoption of health IT systems lags well below the 90 percent threshold the RAND researchers expected by now, a threshold required to demonstrate some of the cost savings and quality improvements cited in its 2005 report. Approximately 40 percent of U.S. physicians and a third of hospitals use a "basic" EHR, and far fewer small practices and small, rural, or nonteaching hospitals utilize them. A much lower percentage use them for anything other than a repository for medical information and to bill insurers.

- Health IT is often difficult to use. The fact is, engineers and IT specialists designed EHRs with little, if any, input from physicians and nurses. So rather than seamlessly integrating into a clinician's workflow the way an iPhone seamlessly integrates into daily life, EHR technologies frequently require that we interrupt our normal workflow for cumbersome, time-consuming tasks that, in our minds, don't make it any easier for us to treat patients.

One surgeon told us that when he logs into his hospital system's EHR, he's confronted with a home screen with 70 icons, including apps for newborn information, pediatric growth charts, and tympanic drawings, none of which he needs. That hardly endears the technology to him.

- The existing fee-for-service reimbursement system provides little incentive to boost efficiency with EHRs. At least one study found that rather than controlling costs, EHRs enable hospitals to boost their reimbursement.[73] As the authors of the RAND report wrote: "Implementing health IT without changing the underlying incentives or delivery processes is unlikely to produce the desired effects on cost, quality, or outcomes."

- EHRs may contribute to medical errors and, potentially, patient harm. Recent studies find that clinicians often override alarms when using computerized prescribing due to "alert fatigue," cut and paste information without reviewing it, and "autofill" information.[74-77]

"Like so many other things in health care, the amount of accomplishment [with EHRs] is well short of the amount of cheerleading."[78]

Mark V. Pauly,
Professor of Health Management at the Wharton School at the University of Pennsylvania,
Interview with *The New York Times*

It's no wonder, then, that even with the more than $6.5 billion that the federal government has handed out so far to encourage EHR adoption through the Health Information Technology for Economic and Clinical Health (HITECH) Act, uptake has been slow. Professionals in other industries just don't get it. Who would turn down money so they can still line their offices with walls of paper files?

Yet, without that pot of promised gold, most of us believe it would be another 30 years or more before our behind-the-times industry finally gave up its horse-and-buggy method of managing data and jumped onto the virtual highway.

So no, we're not where we need to be. But we're farther along than we would have been without HITECH.

"For an EHR to be successful, there must be a top-down culture of using IT to make patient outcomes a priority."

Geeta Nayyar, M.D., MBA
Chief Medical Information Officer,
PatientPoint

What About the Platform?

The platform upon which the mHealth world resides is of utmost importance. Within hospitals and other healthcare facilities, we believe that an "open developer ecosystem" similar to the ones Apple and Google provide is ideal.

Such a system must incorporate all aspects of the healthcare facility/office, from the EHR to the billing system to patient portals and cloud-based data storage so the right individuals at the right time in the right place can share and access the right information.

What About the Platform?

This environment should also allow patients, clinicians, and administrators to securely collect data regardless of where that data originates. We're not there yet, but this is the direction in which we are moving and must continue to move.

Physicians and Tablets: A Match Made in the Apple Store

Physicians may not be crazy about workstation EHRs, but they love their tablets. The portability, long battery life, and small footprint have doctors (and nurses) clamoring to use their tablets as part of patient care. As well they should. Apps that can deliver real-time data from wireless devices at the patient's bedside can provide more relevant clinical information and improve productivity.

For instance, obstetricians at Texas Health Resources, a Dallas-based healthcare system, use the FDA-approved AirStrip app to remotely monitor fetal heart beats, while hospitalists can get EKG readings that they can enlarge and zoom in on from their tablets or smartphones.

In hospitals and freestanding surgical centers owned by Nashville-based HCA, a similar program slashed the average time clinicians spent entering vital signs into the EHR from 41 minutes using a paper-based approach to 23 seconds using the app.[79]

At HCA, physicians also use their iPads to check their daily schedules before heading to the office; receive patient status updates for hospitalized patients; review X-rays and EKGs; educate patients and family members about conditions; and calculate stroke risk and anticoagulant safety for individual patients.

Here at the Cleveland Clinic, where we have more than 1 million square feet in our hospital, our emergency medical team members use tablets to remotely access patient data as they race throughout the hospital during emergencies. This enables them to arrive at the patient's bedside already aware of the patient's vital signs, allergies, clinical notes, and even radiology images. This, in turn, enables medical staff to intervene more quickly, reducing the

Physicians and Tablets: A Match Made in the Apple Store

likelihood that the patient will require more intensive—and expensive—care. It also reduces the risk that the patient will get worse or even die.

The Challenge: Keep It Simple, Stupid

The "EHR dilemma" highlights several lessons for anyone developing any health-related IT software or hardware. The most important: Do it *with*—not *to*—the end users. The doctor, nurse, and patient must work with IT professionals on the design of a program or system *from the beginning.* They should work collaboratively to seek a common understanding of both the problem that needs to be addressed and the capabilities of the IT tools that are available.

Doctors and nurses don't care about bits and bytes, computing power, or code. They care that the technology integrates seamlessly into their workflow with demonstrated improvement in productivity and quality. Medical professionals *are* open to change if it makes sense and if they are empowered to be part of guiding that change. But, if the technology requires that they change how they're used to working and they don't understand why or feel any ownership or influence, it will likely fail.

This back-and-forth approach leads to better results and more robust adoption. We can also say from previous experience that it is a lot of fun!

"When doctors and nurses see that they are in the driver's seat, you don't encounter the behavioral hurdles [to adoption] that otherwise occur."

Axel Nemetz,
Vodafone mHealth Solutions

Keys to successfully engaging providers in mHealth include:

- **Keep it simple.** How easy is it to text on your smartphone? To check the weather on your tablet? To pay your bills online? That's how easy it should be for clinicians to manage their patients' health online. The systems and apps must be intuitive, elegant, and user-friendly. That means clicking *once* to access information, not diving through eight templates.

- **Don't overpromise.** That new diabetes app is not going to cure diabetes in our patients. Nor will accessing patient MRI scans on our tablet free up 10 hours a week. Set realistic expectations so we're not disappointed or frustrated.

- **Show us, don't tell us.** We're scientists. We live and breathe data. So simply telling us that an app will improve patient care and productivity doesn't cut it. Just as with a new drug that comes on the market, we want to see real data from well-designed studies. We need studies like the ones from WellDoc, or the one published in the *Annals of Internal Medicine* in 2012 that showed an EHR *could* improve outcomes in patients with diabetes.[80]

Ponder This ...

Even though EHRs have been around for more than 20 years, their growing pervasiveness in brick-and-mortar systems as well as in the virtual world raises some interesting issues we should consider:

- Who is liable for adverse events or patient deaths if they can be traced back to a software issue?

- How does the EHR interface change how clinicians diagnose and manage patients? As Deborah Burger, president of the California Nurses Association, told a *New York Times* reporter in 2012, while the drop-down menus of "so-called best practices" that EHRs offer can be helpful, "each patient is an individual. We need the ability to change that care plan, based on age and sex and other factors."[78]

- If the software, technology, or interface has not been completely tested and validated before widespread use, are we intentionally exposing patients to harm? Could it be considered, as a *New York Times* article suggested, an "experimental treatment"?[78]

- Where do you get information about your patients when the system crashes, the power goes out for an extended time, or the data is hacked?

- How are modifications, updates, and content management handled within a deployment of an EHR? How are these changes governed in an organization? Are those in charge free of any conflict of interests?

Going mobile? Ask these same questions.

Unintended Consequences from EHRs and mHealth

Eventually, payers, including the federal government (think Medicare), will require that all providers use EHRs and use them for more than data storage. When they do, they need to be aware of the potential for unintended consequences. For instance, we've always assumed that giving patients access to their medical records online and allowing email communication with healthcare providers would reduce healthcare utilization. Yet a 2012 *JAMA* study found just the opposite: patients with such access actually demonstrated *increased* in-person and telephone clinical services for chronic and acute conditions.[81]

We also assume that greater use of technology means fewer medical errors and adverse events. Yet, an Agency for Healthcare Research and Quality (AHRQ) report estimated that if all healthcare providers fully adopted EHRs, the systems could be involved in about 60,000 adverse events a year.[82] Another AHRQ report found that workflow changes related to the EHR "affected interactions, communication, or the relationships between providers and patients," and not in a good way.[83]

The Institute of Medicine (IOM) warned in 2011 of potential risks with health information technology even while admitting that studies on its ability to improve patient safety were mixed. For instance, some studies find fewer medication-related adverse events with the technology; others do not. Same with EHRs.[84]

A major issue that health providers need to consider, the report noted, is the design of their systems. "Case reports suggest that poorly designed health IT can create new hazards in the already complex delivery of care. Although the magnitude of the risk associated with health IT is not known, [examples include] dosing errors, failure to detect life-threatening illnesses, and delaying treatment due to poor human–computer interactions or loss of data," which have led to serious injury and death.[84]

AHRQ is trying to address these risks with an application designed to identify, communicate, and track potential and actual hazards associated with health IT.[82] This "proactive hazard control" offers several advantages, an AHRQ report noted:

- It broadens the focus from one on safety incidents to a systematic focus on the full range of hazards that health IT and its interactions with healthcare systems may create.

- It expands the typical focus on "user error" to a holistic view of how clinicians, health IT vendors, and local IT implementers unknowingly create hazards.

- It engages the skills and passion for quality of the most knowledgeable stakeholders: clinicians, patients, safety teams, healthcare informaticians, and IT business analysts, trainers, and production-support teams.

- It enables analysis of potential hazards in a non-emergent, less stressful environment, which increases the likelihood of identifying unanticipated hazards.

- It reduces important forms of bias associated with retrospective analysis, particularly hindsight, political, sponsor, and confirmation biases.

- It can potentially improve the quality and efficiency of patient care while enhancing public trust.

- It can reduce the number of expensive emergency fixes required after hazards are identified retrospectively and care is already compromised.

The end result will likely be new reporting mechanisms for vendors and users to report health IT-related deaths, serious injuries, or unsafe conditions similar to the FDA's Adverse Event Reporting System.[84]

The reality is that we don't really know what the overall affect of mHealth will be on productivity, patient safety, and cost. What we *do* know from the EHR experiment is that the technology itself is not a panacea. We still need studies that examine outcomes from using mHealth and EHRs. We also need to adapt our study methodologies so that useful data is published in a timely manner. Many randomized studies take several years from start to publication. By then, many mHealth-related technologies will have moved on, given the lightning-fast pace of innovation.

And, obviously, we need to create safer systems. This, the IOM report warned, "begins with user-centered design principles." Human factor engineering is an essential step in the development of mHealth solutions. Understanding not only the technology, but how it impacts, interacts, and alters the care ecosystem are important considerations as we embrace this new technology.

Such systems should also:

- Undergo adequate testing and quality assurance assessments in actual and/or simulated clinical environments, with system designers and users working together,

- Provide easy retrieval of accurate, timely, and reliable data,

- Incorporate simple and intuitive data displays,

- Yield evidence at the point of care to inform decisions,

- Enhance workflow, perhaps by automating mundane tasks or streamlining work, without increasing physical or cognitive workloads,

- Allow easy transfer of information to and from other organizations and providers,

- Cause no unanticipated downtime.

All of which is to say is that if we want to avoid the minefields and missed opportunities of that first troubled romance with digital technology—the EHR—we need to take the IOM's advice to heart with every mHealth app, device, and system we design and implement.

What System Do We Need?

Looking to mobilize your practice? Answer these questions first:

1. **What do we want the system to do?** Allow patients to make their own appointments and email their providers? Enable us to take advantage of government incentives? Provide a patient portal for virtual visits? Make it easier to document care provided and identify care needed?

2. **Will this fit with our workflow and care environment?**

What System Do We Need?

Here is where many earlier systems failed—they were desktop-based. You need a truly mobile, possibly cloud-based system that enables you to take notes, capture data, and take action no matter where you are or what device you're using.

3. **Is it compliant with the federal Health Insurance Portability and Accountability Act (HIPAA)?** You're subject to major fines if it isn't.

4. **How secure is it?** This means more than passwords. It may mean biometrics for access, differing levels of access depending on the individual (should your receptionist have access to patient charts?), and automatic log-off systems. Some systems enable data to be remotely deleted from the hard drive if the computer, smartphone, or tablet is lost or stolen. You also need a security policy. (We cover these topics in more detail in Chapter 2.)

5. **What kind of training and ongoing support is available?** Medicine doesn't keep business hours. You need support 24/7.

6. **How flexible is the software for updating as the technology changes?** The last thing you want is for new regulatory requirements or clinical evidence to come along and knock your system out of the lineup.

7. **Can the system interact with other entities such as hospitals, skilled nursing facilities, and pharmacies?** Coordination of care, accountable care organizations (ACOs), and medical homes all require that digital systems talk to one another and share information.

Getting Specific: mHealth and Patient Engagement

As we've said many times before, the shifting sands of health care require that we toss aside more than 100 years of history and move into a new paradigm, which many of us are still defining. That shift is coming, in a large part, from the outside, as payers, employers, and patients push us to change.

The push comes through value-based purchasing, ever-increasing quality benchmarks, new care models such as ACOs and medical homes, and reimbursement "carrots" and "sticks" tied to the outcomes of the care we deliver.

We could write an entire book on where mHealth fits into just those four areas (and maybe we will), but for now we want to highlight one area as particularly relevant to providers: patient engagement.

mHealth Cuts Time to Treatment for Stroke Patients

When patients are having a stroke, minutes matter. Doctors have up to four-and-a-half hours to start clot-busting treatment with tissue plasminogen activator (tPA), and one of the gold standards of quality in stroke treatment is a door-to-needle (DTN) time of just 60 minutes.

Hospitals that need to improve their time should consider text messaging. A study from University of California, San Francisco, researchers presented at the 2013 American Academy of Neurology meeting found that using a real-time text messaging system to assemble the stroke team when patients were on their way to or entered the ED dramatically improved DTN time compared to the traditional paging system.

The researchers compared times between 95 acute ischemic stroke patients under the paging system and 46 under the texting system. Half the patients in the texting cohort received tPA within 60 minutes versus 16 percent of those in the paging cohort, a highly significant difference.[85]

Tools Supporting the Patient

Patient engagement is a cornerstone of U.S. healthcare reform. It calls for patients to partner with their healthcare providers in their care and for providers to encourage such engagement. This concept is a key part of initiatives such as medical homes and ACOs.

There is good evidence that promoting such engagement results in improved quality and lower costs. Motivated patients make better day-to-day health decisions, are more likely to keep appointments, tend to be more satisfied with their care, experience fewer complications, and have improved quality of life.[86-88]

The U.S. government has embedded patient engagement within the meaningful use requirements healthcare entities must meet to receive incentive payments for EHR implementation. There are three stages, two of which have been implemented and all of which require patient engagement.

In Stage 2 requirements, more than half of all patients in a practice must have timely online access to their health information, including diagnostic test results, medication lists, and discharge instructions. They must be able to download and transmit such information and have bidirectional secure email with their clinicians. Stage 3 is expected to require that patients be able to input data directly into their EHR.[42]

Obviously, the EHR is an important component of patient engagement. But hospitals and healthcare providers know they must go further if they are to meet all of the quality standards required today. mHealth provides an important option.

A variety of studies find that putting apps and other technologies into patients' hands to collect information about their health status, communicate it to physicians, and receive information improves outcomes and costs.[89] As the chief technology and information officer at the Robert Wood Johnson Foundation wrote: "When you make it easy for people to capture information from their lives and share it with clinicians, they feel empowered to take a more active role in their health—and this engagement can lead to better outcomes."[89] This can also improve productivity as providers "offload" certain tasks to patients.[90]

Here are just a handful of the thousands of apps, programs, and devices that can improve patient engagement:

Interactive whiteboards. Sharp Memorial Hospital in San Diego was one of the first hospitals in the nation to install the GetWellNetwork's Interactive Patient Whiteboard in all patient rooms. The system uses the in-room television as a central communication tool between patients, families, and care team members so they can share information on everything from daily care plans to medications, vital signs, schedules, and discharge planning.

"It turns the TV into an extension of the healthcare team," said Susan Stone, Sharp's vice president of patient care and chief nursing officer. It also provides education about the patient's condition, quizzes designed to test their knowledge of the information and assess their readiness for discharge, and safety videos on topics like infection control and fall awareness.

The system stresses the role the patient plays as an integral part of the care team and even allows patients to designate a family member or friend as part of that team. The "whiteboard" also includes identification information, expected length of stay, summary of tests, procedures, the "plan of the day," and a column in which patients or their family members can leave questions and notes for the healthcare team.

"This is really activating the patient and getting them to interact with their information and understand their health condition," said Stone. "We understand that the patient is the team leader, and we are facilitating their team leader status by enabling them to take control of their own health." The more information patients have, she said, the more likely they are to get engaged.

So how does the hospital ensure patients use the system? Simple: they can't use the "real" TV until they view the mandatory welcome and safety videos.

Patient engagement systems (PES). These systems collect all patient information into one mobile portal linked to the EHR to deliver patient-centric clinical decision support to physicians based on clinical findings and provide personalized messages to patients about those care plans.[91] Studies evaluating their impact on patients with diabetes found they significantly reduced hospital admissions and charges, as well as ED utilization and charges.[92] A PES can also improve the provision of guideline-recommended care to patients, and, in one study, resulted in average savings of $3,563 per patient by the fourth year of use.[93,94]

EmmiTransition. This system triggers automated phone calls that ask patients with congestive heart failure (CHF) to assess their weight and other clinical indicators, then email the results to physicians who identify any "red flags." Patients enrolled in the program showed significantly reduced readmission rates (from approximately 20 percent to less than 6 percent). "This helped us improve interactions with patients," said Louis Teichholz, M.D., medical director of cardiac services at Hackensack University Medical Center, which piloted the program. "One of the things with readmission is patient understanding, interaction, and education. We think this helped."[95]

Estrellita. This app enables caregivers of preterm, high-risk infants to collect information on the baby's fussiness, diapering, and weight, as well as information on their own stress levels and indicators for postpartum depression. A healthcare provider receives the information and remotely monitors caregivers and babies for signs of trouble. The manufacturer hopes to expand the app to low-income countries.[91]

Better Day Health. This Web-based app uses voice recognition at the point of care to make patient notes immediately available to physicians and patients and enable patients to provide their own input into the record.[91]

BreathEasy. This asthma app captures and reports patient observations of daily living (ODLs), including how often they use a controller and rescue medications, symptom levels, quality of life, and smoking. Clinicians receive the information on a Web-based dashboard that lets them quickly assess their patients' status. Patients said it was easy to use, they enjoyed collecting and viewing their ODLs, and they better understood their asthma control and triggers. Clinicians said the information was "not overwhelming," provided clinically useful information, and led to patient education opportunities, therapy escalation, and changed diagnoses.[96]

Opening Pandora's Box?

There's just one problem with the push toward patient engagement with mHealth. It scares the hell out of a lot of doctors.

Research from PwC and *The Economist* found that 42 percent of physicians are worried that mHealth will make their patients too independent, with 53 percent of those who were practicing less than five years expressing this concern.[97] Just a third encourage their patients to use mHealth applications to take a greater role in managing their health, while 13 percent (24 percent of younger physicians) actively discourage this. Resistance exists even in emerging countries.

Physicians fear that putting more power into the hands of patients will reduce their own authority and even the need for doctors. Indeed, the PwC/*Economist* survey found that if patients reap the improved control over their health expected from mHealth, it would lead to a "substantial, disruptive move away from doctor-directed care towards a patient-as-consumer model."[97]

A session presented at the 2012 mHealth Summit in Washington, D.C., titled "In the Future, Doctors May Not Always Be Human," took that paradigm a step further when presenters questioned the need for "human" doctors at all. Vinod Khosla, cofounder and CEO of Sun Microsystems, contended that just as a computer bested a human in chess 16 years ago, so, too, can the ability of today's computers to "learn" best the cognitive limitations and biases of today's medical professionals.

His copresenter, Joseph Kvedar, M.D., founder and director of the Center for Connected Health in Boston, predicted that given the pending shortage of doctors, computers *have* to be utilized more for the routine tasks that make up so much of a doctor's day, including charting and even reviewing discharge or medication instructions with patients. As for the patient perspective on the "robotization of medicine"? Patients prefer it for some things, he said, since they can take as much time as they want and ask as many questions as they want without embarrassment.

We address patient engagement in more detail in the next chapter.

"[mHealth] changes the balance of power. It is not surprising that doctors would be concerned."

Steinar Pedersen,

Chief Executive Officer
Tromsø Telemedicine Consult[97]

Way Cool: JiffPad

JiffPad enables healthcare providers to use their iPads to provide patient education in the office, then preserves all the instructions and background information into a HIPAA-compliant digital file that can be emailed to patients for viewing in a secure patient portal. Providers purchase the $99 app, not patients.[98]

Conquering High Readmission Rates with mHealth

In 2012, the U.S. Centers for Medicare & Medicaid Services (CMS) began penalizing hospitals for readmissions within 30 days for patients with CHF, chronic obstructive pulmonary disease (COPD), or pneumonia. That list will significantly increase in the coming years, as will the financial penalties. So, hospitals are scrambling to reduce their 30-day readmission rates, which are about 20 percent for all Medicare patients, far higher for those three conditions.[99,100]

One option? Remote monitoring, also called tele-homecare, telecare, and even telemedicine. Patients or caregivers provide daily updated medical data from home, these days mainly using a computer, cellphone, or wireless device. The data is fed to nurses or other healthcare providers at a central location who review it and flag any warning signs of problems for follow-up.[101]

For instance, a U.S. Department of Veterans Affairs (VA) hospital in Gainesville, Fla., used telemonitoring to slash its readmission rate for heart failure patients and inpatient lengths of stay by half, as well as reduce unscheduled primary care clinic visits.[102]

Other examples:

- Massachusetts General Hospital randomized 150 recently hospitalized patients with CHF to either usual post-discharge care or a remote monitoring system for six months. Patients transmitted their vital signs data to a nurse who shared any potential problems with a physician. Those in the remote monitoring group had a lower all-cause and heart failure-related readmission rate (0.64 versus 0.73), although the difference was not statistically significant. However, the study was not powered to demonstrate reductions in readmissions, but to assess its feasibility.[20]

All participants said the equipment was simple and easy to use and that they felt they had greater control of their health. Most also thought that the program should continue longer. Since the pilot trial, all Partners hospitals in Boston implemented the program, which was modified to include a shared portal to improve communication between the nurse and care team, increased use of orders that allow the nurse to make timely treatment changes approved by the doctor, physician champions to promote the program among their colleagues, a patient video to help patients understand the program and hear from past participants, and an opt-out system for enrollment.

- Texas Health Resources reduced its heart failure readmissions by a third, from 14 percent to 10 percent, with an AT&T program that remotely monitors CHF patients for 90 days after hospital discharge. Patients receive vital sign monitors to track their weight, pulse, and blood pressure; tablets to input the data; and apps that link their data to their EHR.[103]

- Geisinger Health System's monitoring program combines an interactive voice response protocol telemonitoring system with case management to reduce emergency department visits and readmissions. A study involving 875 Medicare Advantage patients enrolled in the program compared to 2,420 matched control patients who only received case management found that the combination of monitoring and case management reduced 30-day readmissions 44 percent compared to the case management–only group.[104]

- A Danish study evaluating the impact of telemedicine video consultations between hospital-based respiratory nurses and recently discharged patients found a significant reduction in the number of patients readmitted (12 percent in the intervention group and 22 percent in the control group), with high patient satisfaction.[105]

Clearly, mHealth, whether in the form of telemonitoring, apps, video consultations, or other approaches, offers a significant opportunity to reduce the frustratingly high rate of 30-day hospital readmissions.

Telemedicine: Beyond Readmissions

Telemedicine is about more than preventing readmissions. It's also about bringing physician services to remote areas, whether in developed or developing countries; providing access to specialists from other institutions; streamlining healthcare delivery; and even improving reimbursement and quality of life for doctors.

For instance, a company called Teladoc partners with health insurers to provide telehealth options for their employees. Doctors, all of whom are board certified in their specialties, log into the system from anywhere they have a computer and provide online consults—for which they are paid without any third-party reimbursement hassles—any time they want.

In Kentucky, primary care physician William "Chuck" Thornbury, M.D., created a service that allows doctors to conduct house calls via their smartphones. Each "Me-Visit" costs patients about $32 and is available 24 hours a day. Results from a University of Kentucky study found that most patients preferred the e-visit to an in-person visit. Most visits were conducted after hours, 90 percent of those before 9 p.m.

After two years, Dr. Thornbury estimated that the e-visits increased his rural practice's capacity to see patients by 15 percent, with a similar per-patient reduction in costs. Rolled out nationally, he estimates it could put a significant dent in the $9 billion a year now spent on after-hours care, much of which is provided in higher-cost urgent care centers and EDs.[106]

The Challenge: Demonstrating a Return on Investment

Health systems and providers need to see a return on their investment in mHealth. This return can be related to quality, safety, satisfaction, financial performance, or some combination of all four. In our experience, this is quite possible—if done the right way.

For instance, a study published in the journal *Circulation: Cardiovascular Quality and Outcomes* evaluated a telestroke program among eight hospitals. In this type of system, neurologists and other specialists at a stroke-certified or accredited hospital (the "hub") provide remote guidance for hospitals without those resources (the "spokes"). In this study, seven "spoke" hospitals and one "hub" hospital saved about $358,435 a year altogether. The spoke hospitals reaped the actual savings—$109,080 each—and the hub hospital bore all the cost, $405,121, but cost sharing would eliminate that disparity and allow all the hospitals to realize savings.[107]

In addition, the system resulted in 45 more patients per year treated with tPA and 20 more with endovascular stroke therapies compared to patients in hospitals without such a network. It also prevented 114 admissions to the hub hospital and resulted in an estimated six additional home discharges.

A study in the journal *Health Affairs* found significant cost savings from a CMS demonstration project called Health Buddy. The intervention involved patients with diabetes, COPD, or CHF. Patients used a handheld device at home to enter responses to diagnosis-specific questions about their symptoms, vital signs, self-management knowledge, and health behavior. Their responses were uploaded to a Web-based computer application that stratified their responses based on risk and alerted care managers to patients requiring intervention. The care managers followed up by telephone.[108]

About 1,700 Medicare patients used the system. Cost analysis comparing before-and-after costs for those patients and a matched control group found that quarterly mean spending in the study group dropped between $312 and $542 per person (between 7.7 percent and 13.3 percent) over two years, compared with that of the control group. Factoring in the average cost of the program ($120 a month the first year, $128 a month the third year) still resulted in net savings of between 4.3 percent and 9.8 percent.

At Dartmouth-Hitchcock Medical Center in Lebanon, N.H., postsurgical remote monitoring with pulse oximetry and clinician notification technologies saved an estimated $1.5 million in one year on just one floor, thanks to fewer transfers to the intensive care unit, as well as significantly reducing lengths of stay and mortality rates.[109]

Meanwhile, a study from Pennsylvania State University in College Station found a whopping 62.5 percent drop in hospitalization costs for diabetes patients who received home monitoring compared to those who did not.[110]

Figure 3-1 demonstrates a model of the potential savings of a small, integrated healthcare network over five years using home telehealth for patients with CHF.

Figure 3-1. Potential Savings of Telehealth for Small, Integrated Healthcare Network Over 5 Years

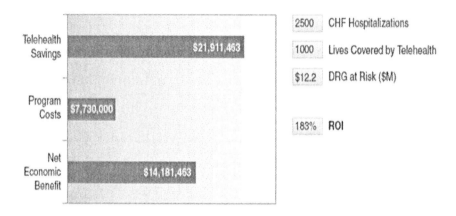

Source: Honeywell HomMed. Telehealth for Chronic Care Management

Implemented properly, for the right reasons and with the right patients, mHealth has the potential to "bend the curve," providing much-needed cost savings and slowing the steep upward trajectory of healthcare costs in the United States and other countries.

Way Cool: Preventive Services Selector

The U.S.-based Agency for Healthcare Research and Quality is getting into the app business. Its Electronic Preventive Services Selector (ePSS) tool for iPhones enables healthcare providers to search for up-to-date recommendations of the U.S. Preventive Services Task Force based on a patient's individual characteristics or risk factors, such as age, gender, tobacco use, and sexual activity.

Way Cool: Preventive Services Selector

Recommended preventive services are given one of five grades ranging from A (highly recommend) to I (insufficient evidence to make a recommendation). The app garnered a five-star rating in the iTunes store in 2012.

Rounding in Real Time

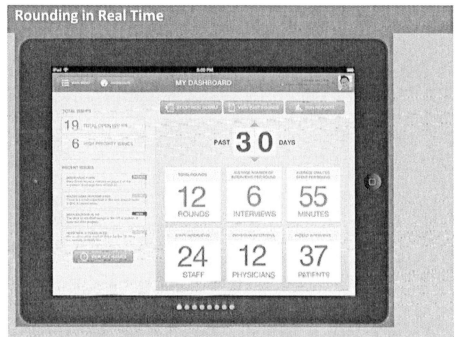

My Rounding Dashboard

We think of rounding as something clinicians do each morning on their hospitalized patients. But hospital administrators also need to "round" to keep their fingers on the pulse of their institution, both anecdotally and quantitatively. That's where My Rounding, an iPad app that provides a real-time option for managers to collect data on specific issues, comes in.

"Rounding on all levels of employees, from floor nurses to physicians, as well as patients, creates a culture of continuing improvement and open communication," said Dave Marshall, a principle and cofounder of Colorado-based MyRounding Solutions, which develops, markets, and sells technology solutions for hospitals and healthcare organizations to perform

Rounding in Real Time

structured leadership rounding and replace paper-based methods.

The iPad app the company developed enables managers to enter data as they see it, providing "real time" information, as well as immediate analytics on a dashboard that allows for customized reports. The administrators ask a series of scripted questions, such as, "What is preventing you from delivering the best care you can?" then enters the answer into the app. "They develop a mini gap analysis on the spot," said Marshall.

In addition, executives collect information on employees who deserve special recognition.

The value-added reward for the hospital comes in reducing paperwork and staff time required to enter such data into computer systems, Marshall said. Other advantages are the standardized questions, real-time data, and flexibility to change the questions on a daily—or even hourly—basis.

Chapter 3: Key Takeaways

✓ The current business model in health care is massive and challenging but can properly support and nurture mHealth development and deployment.

✓ As we plan for mHealth, we should embrace the lessons that have been learned from EHR implementation. The "EHR Dilemma" cannot be solved, but it can be managed. Let's learn from the past, make "new" mistakes when we do mHealth, and then learn from that experience as well.

✓ mHealth applications can demonstrate improved quality of care and reduced costs—if implemented appropriately.

✓ Clinician buy-in requires systems and apps that are simple to use, integrate seamlessly into the workflow, and demonstrate validated outcomes.

✓ mHealth acceptance relies not on intuitive deductions about its clinical and economic potential, but on the outcomes of quality studies designed to objectively evaluate that potential.

Chapter 4. mHealth and the Patient: A Perfect Match?

"The patient of tomorrow is the biggest switch. People need to take ownership. They need to seize the moment and seize the data. The new medicine is plugged into you. It's understanding you, which we've never really done before, and you drive it. You've got the data and you've got information that you never had before. Wouldn't you like that information? Most people would. And wouldn't you like to be helping to call the shots?"

Eric Topol, M.D.
Professor of Genomics
The Scripps Research Institute—2013 interview on NBC's *Rock Center*

Would you choose a bank that didn't give you daily access to your account information, let you pay your bills online, provide a national network of ATMs, or allow deposits with your smartphone? Probably not.

So why do medical professionals expect consumers to choose physicians and health networks that maintain inconvenient office hours, don't provide online access to our medical records, and don't communicate electronically?

These providers, who don't offer the kinds of service and mobile accessibility we have come to expect from other retail and service interactions, may soon find themselves with empty waiting rooms. "I fired my doctor because I couldn't communicate with him via email—couldn't even leave a voice mail for him," one patient told us. "I couldn't schedule appointments online, and, despite the fact that he used an electronic medical record, I had no access to my own data."

Welcome to the "consumerization" of health care. More and more, we want—no, we demand—that accessing the healthcare system be as easy and transparent as ordering books, planning a vacation, or paying a credit card bill online. We want our data available across platforms when we want it, not when it's convenient for the physician's office or hospital to provide it. We want to know how much a procedure will cost, how well the physician (or hospital) does that procedure, and how often they've done it.

We want to see the results of our chest X-rays, including the images themselves, on our cellphones, as well as send emails to our physicians and book follow-up appointments, all without having to leave messages, navigate voice mail, or play phone tag. We want our transactional experiences to be completely mobile.

A poll from Wolters Kluwer Health released in November 2012 found that 80 percent of the 1,000 U.S. adults surveyed viewed the "consumerization" of health care as a good thing. Three-fourths said they felt prepared to make their own healthcare decisions, including researching treatment options. About half told pollsters that taking control of their health care makes them feel more empowered and better about the quality of care they receive.[87]

In addition, 40 percent said that, assuming similar experience and quality, they were most likely to choose a more "technologically advanced" physician. They defined "technologically advanced" as the ability to communicate via email, schedule appointments online, and use mobile devices or computers during office visits.[87]

Other research finds that patients with poorly managed medical conditions are more likely to use mHealth if they don't have to bear the cost themselves.[97]

Meanwhile, a 2012 study from The Economist Intelligence Unit that was commissioned by the consulting firm PwC found that in the next three years, about half of consumers expect mHealth to change how they seek information on health issues; receive general healthcare information from providers; manage their overall health, chronic conditions, and medication; communicate with their healthcare providers; and measure and share their vital health information (Figure 4-1).

Figure 4-1. Potential Savings of Telehealth for Small, Integrated Healthcare Network Over 5 Years

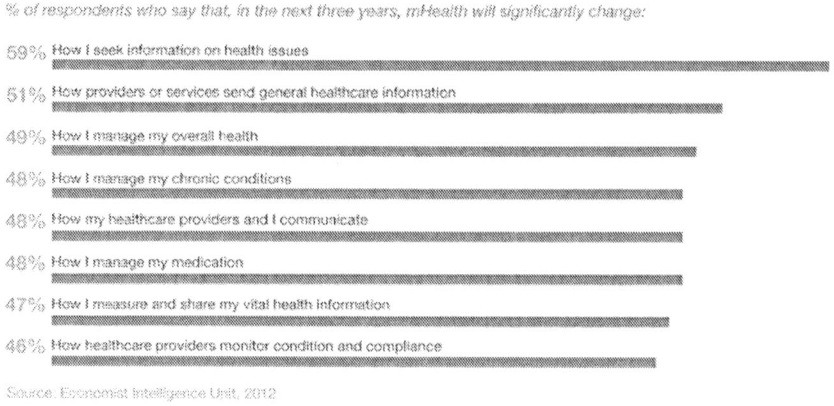

% of respondents who say that, in the next three years, mHealth will significantly change:

59% How I seek information on health issues

51% How providers or services send general healthcare information

49% How I manage my overall health

48% How I manage my chronic conditions

48% How my healthcare providers and I communicate

48% How I manage my medication

47% How I measure and share my vital health information

46% How healthcare providers monitor condition and compliance

Source: Economist Intelligence Unit, 2012

Source: PwC analysis based on Economist Intelligence Unit research, 2012.

Nearly half also expected mHealth to change how their providers monitor their conditions and adherence to management recommendations.[97] The main reasons patients want to use or increase usage of mHealth applications and services, however, is to access their healthcare providers more conveniently and effectively; reduce their own healthcare costs; and "take greater control" over their own health, a huge step in the direction of empowering and engaging patients. And a huge step toward achieving the vision of "accountable care."

What's happening throughout health care is what happened in maternity wards in the 1980s when women became consumers, not just patients, and demanded a birthing "experience." Hospitals gave it to them, adding luxurious birthing suites, labor and delivery classes, and breastfeeding support, and allowing partners and others into the delivery room.

Today, however, in addition to soft lighting, wood floors, and comfy chairs, hospitals must give those women the ability to register online, take a virtual tour of the maternity floor, track pregnancy and labor on their smartphones, email or text their doctors for appointments and when labor begins, and invite their families to participate virtually in the birth via a hospital-provided webcam.

And that's just the tip of the proverbial iceberg.

Why Do Patients Want mHealth?

- Access my healthcare providers more conveniently/effectively
- Reduce my own healthcare costs
- Maintain greater control over my own health
- Gain easy access to information that is difficult or impossible for me to obtain from other sources
- Get better quality health care

Patient-Centered Care: The New Paradigm

"There is huge potential here, but you need to get off the Web and into the patients' pocket[s]. You also need to give the patient real value. Not having to repeat your meds to a doctor isn't real value. If people think it is, they don't understand value from a patient's perspective."

John Gomez,
CEO, Sensato,
Interview with HISTalk, September 19, 2011

Patient-centered and patient-directed health care represents a paradigm shift from a healthcare system that often seems centered on the provider to one that consistently puts the patient first.

As we highlighted in the previous chapter, our healthcare system, as currently designed, often creates situations in which providers talk *to* patients, rather than *with* them; blame patients when treatments fail; have little expectation or trust that patients will participate in their own care; and exhibit little patience with patients who question the provider's approach, research their own conditions, or ask for more time or information. Providers and patients alike are frustrated by these circumstances.

Healthcare reform is built on the assumption that this *can* and *should* change. New delivery systems such as patient-centered medical homes and accountable care organizations (see next section titled, *Putting the Patient First*) are designed to provide coordinated care with the patient at the center.

This is about much more than creating a better experience for patients. Increasingly, the evidence suggests that this approach produces better *clinical* outcomes. New methods of communicating with patients recognize that engaged patients working collaboratively with providers produce the best results. In one study, researchers randomized 509 patients to care with either family practitioners or internists. After controlling for variables such as gender, age, weight, and health status, the researchers found that those who received patient-centered care demonstrated significantly fewer visits to specialists, fewer hospitalizations, and fewer tests. Not surprisingly, they also incurred significantly lower charges during the one-year study.[111]

Table 4-1 depicts today's model of care versus the patient-centered, coordinated approach we're moving toward.

Table 4-1. Provider-Centered vs. Patient-Centered Health Care

Provider Centered	Patient Centered
Fragmented care	Teams of providers that include patients and families
Primary care physician = gatekeeper	Coordinated care across organizations; primary care physician as advocate or coach
Paternalistic care	Patient-centered care
Little focus on data	Information technology critical
Acute-care focused	Preventive and chronic-care focused
Little attention to cost	Focus on value with protocols and practice standards designed to achieve the best outcome for the lowest cost

Many of the mHealth technologies discussed in this chapter move us toward a more patient-centered system by giving patients the control, information, and feedback they need to better manage their own health. After all, if tapping a few keys on your smartphone can tell you at a glance where your blood sugar is heading and provide feedback on what you should do, you're now empowered to take the steps you need to improve it—without waiting for a doctor appointment.

If you can peer into your medical record and see that a test result seems out of whack—but your doctor didn't get back to you about it—you can shoot off a quick email asking what's going on.

In fact, that ability to communicate with your doctor (or care team) when you want and how you want, rather than trying to get through a receptionist and playing phone tag, puts you in the driver's seat.

"mHealth technologies are a valuable partner in health care's shift towards a delivery model that is patient-centered and value-based. Mobile technologies can help to facilitate that shift among clinicians, payers, life sciences companies, and consumers by defining and directing the patient-centered model towards health care that is community-based, integrated, seamless, and assimilated into the daily lives of consumers accustomed to an 'on-demand' environment."

Deloitte Center for Health Solutions.
mHealth in an mWorld: How Mobile Technology Is Transforming Health Care.
2012

Putting the Patient First: The PCMH and ACO

The patient-centered medical home (PCMH) is built on six principles:

1. An ongoing relationship between patient and personal physician

2. A physician-directed (not bureaucratically directed) medical practice

3. A whole-person orientation

4. Coordination and integration of care, quality, and safety

5. Enhanced access to care

6. Payment that recognizes the added value a PCMH provides

The National Committee for Quality Assurance (NCQA) accredits medical homes based on their adherence to more than a dozen requirements. Technically, you can have a PCMH without health information technology (HIT), but realistically we don't think it's possible. You must have an electronic health record (EHR) to track and measure the care provided, interact with patients, and provide patient education. We view the personal health record as essential to enhance accessibility and communication, track referrals and results, schedule appointments, and manage prescription refills, among other tasks.

In an accountable care organization (ACO), various healthcare providers join together to provide the entire continuum of care for patients. This includes primary care clinicians and specialists for outpatient care; hospitals for inpatient care; and skilled nursing facilities and home health agencies for post-acute care. These delivery models partner with PCMHs to provide care within and outside of the primary care setting. While you can have a PCMH without an ACO, it is difficult to imagine an effective ACO that does not include PCMHs.

Reimbursements for these new delivery models vary. One commonly used option is "bundling," where the ACO receives a fixed fee for providing care across the continuum and distributes the fee based on outcomes to those providing the care. Another is "shared savings," in which providers are paid on a fee-for-service basis and receive a percentage of any savings realized under the new model.

Perhaps the biggest challenge is that we currently have two parallel systems in place. The movement from the old, fee-for-service, quantity-based model of payment to the new, value-based model is occurring in a halting and uncoordinated fashion. This is very difficult for organizations to manage, because they must time their changes to match the changing rules. Move too quickly into the new model and they may find that the already slim financial margins of medicine have vanished. Move too slowly and they will not be ready for the massive change and reorganization required to succeed in this new world.

It's a difficult balance. To paraphrase hockey legend Wayne Gretzky: You want to skate to where the puck is going to be ... but not get there before the puck does!

Personal Health Records: The Window into a Patient's Health

"Patient-centered care will be the hallmark of transformation of care. Patients taking responsibility for their own clinical outcomes and wellness is essential to improving care and reducing costs. The centerpiece enabler to patient-centered care is the personal health record and similar portals. This capability empowers the patient with the tools and information they need to be accountable to themselves for the care provided."

Bertram S. Reese,
Senior Vice President and Chief Information Officer,
Sentara Healthcare, Virginia Beach, Virginia

When is an electronic health record a personal health record (PHR)? Although the two terms are often used interchangeably, the answer is clear: When the patient can access and control it. While the EHR is basically an electronic version of the paper medical record populated with information from clinicians, PHRs are interactive portals that allow patients to enter their own data; use that data to trigger personalized health information, reminders, and recommendations; and access health-related coaching and information.[89]

"The power of next-generation PHRs lies in their capacity to be coupled with alerts, reminders and other decision-support tools that help people take action to improve their health or manage their conditions," notes a report from the Robert Wood Johnson Foundation's (RWJF) Project HealthDesign, which funds projects to develop the next-generation PHRs. "By doing this, PHR systems and applications will facilitate information to be shared easily between patients and providers and will become dynamic resources for action."[89]

One goal of Project HealthDesign is to incorporate patient-generated data called "observations of daily living" (ODLs) into the PHR. This includes information such as sleep, diet, exercise, mood, and medication adherence. Such data can provide important information to clinicians about a patient's status and are often more important to patients in terms of assessing how well a treatment is working than the tests and X-rays we rely on.

To that end, project grants encourage organizations to integrate ODLs into the PHR and EHR to improve health decision-making. "The ultimate test for a PHR is not the data it stores, but the actions that result from its use," says David Ahern, Ph.D., national program director for RWJF's Health eTechnologies Initiative.[89]

When they work well, PHRs can improve health. In one study, researchers evaluated the medical records of 10,746 adults with type 2 diabetes who saw their primary care physician at least twice. The goal was to see if there was any correlation between the PHR and quality outcomes. They found that PHR users had significantly better measures on diabetes quality profiles. For instance, they were twice as likely to have their A1C tested, and their most recent result was a third lower than patients who didn't use the PHR. The benefits remained regardless of how often patients used the PHR.[112]

But Will They Share?

A study published in the *Journal of the American Medical Informatics Association* in early 2013, in which researchers asked 30 patients which elements of their EHR data they'd be willing to share, found that more than 75 percent said they'd share their entire EHR with their primary care physician, but most would only share with other healthcare providers if there was no sensitive health data within the record. None would be comfortable sharing their data with health insurers, government agencies, or other non-healthcare providers.[113]

Project HealthDesign also found that patients are more concerned with having flexible and easy access to their health information than they are with privacy. Thus, they are willing to make *some* privacy trade-offs to access their medical data as easily as they access their banking information.

"A lot of the emphasis in health care technology is still on the clinician and what's happening inside the hospital and the clinic. We're moving that discussion into the patient's household."

Patricia Flatley Brennan, R.N., Ph.D.,
National Program Director,
Project HealthDesign

Sadly, the Wolters Kluwer survey discussed in the beginning of this chapter found that just 20 percent of those surveyed had access to a PHR.[114]

That's something healthcare executives like Marcy Mishiwiec, R.N., who directs Entity Support Services at Sharp HealthCare in San Diego, Calif., is trying to change. Sharp was one of the first health systems in the country to implement a PHR, and today about a third of its patients use it.

MySharp links patients to the EHR and allows patients to securely email their physicians or nurses, make appointments online, and review test results. It also provides a health profile to patients consisting of their most recent vital signs (e.g., weight, blood pressure, allergies, immunizations) and enables them to print an immunization record, make online requests for information, and assign proxies to view their health records. Because Sharp is a vertically integrated system, patients can also access their pharmacy information and order refills through their PHR.

Setting up a PHR isn't as easy as simply opening up the EHR to the patient, Mishiwiec warns. You have to consider issues such as who will have access. Is it just the patient or can they grant access to other people? How about teenagers? Can they prevent their parents/guardians from accessing it? *What* can patients access? For instance, should they be able to read the clinical and progress notes? And how will you verify (and protect) the patient's identity and information?

You also have to consider not just the federal Health Insurance Portability and Accountability Act, or HIPAA, but state laws governing privacy and the release of medical information. For instance, in California, lab results that may indicate a malignancy— even a questionable Pap test—can't be released electronically or via email. Patients looking for that information will see, instead, a note that if they haven't received an update via mail, they should contact their doctor. Most PHR systems, however, don't release results until the doctor has reviewed them.

Time to Change the Paradigm?

The current approach with PHRs is primarily about extending access *to* patients. But what if we flipped that paradigm on its head? What if we put the patient in the center and made the patient the master of this information ecosystem, letting the *patient* decide which healthcare providers get access to the PHR? What if all data flowed automatically to the patient's PHR (it is their data after all!)? This model would truly put patients in the driver's seat and might accelerate the changes we need in our healthcare system.

No matter how good the PHR, it doesn't work if patient doesn't use it. Sharp found the most effective way to get patients to sign up for PHRs is to have their physicians recommend it, then allow patients to sign up in the office with the help of the office staff. The registration process must be quick, easy, and intuitive, Mishiwiec said. Today, Sharp patients can sign up in as little as two minutes. About a third of those in the outpatient setting have registered, a rate considered quite high in the industry.

At the Cleveland Clinic, we adopted an even more aggressive stance. All patients seen in our clinics automatically have their PHRs activated. This opt-out model has remarkably improved our utilization and adoption.

But even this is not enough. As we gain experience with patient portals and PHRs, it is increasingly clear that the real goal should not be just registering the patient, but creating an active, engaged patient.

The most effective approaches recognize that patients will move through stages of adoption: from awareness, to activation (signing up), to active engagement. Thus, we need to create processes linked to the PHR that make them "sticky," bringing patients to the PHR several times a week in much the same way they check their weather app or Facebook account.

That means the PHR must be part of a mobile experience that goes beyond emailing the doctor. You should be able to gather just-in-time data when an event occurs. If you feel dizzy, you should be able to go to your PHR and rate the dizziness and enter when it occurred and what you were doing. This is information that will help the physician in diagnosis and treatment. Similarly, you should enter your weight into the PHR once a week and, in return, immediately view a chart tracking your weight over time. It should include a food diary and exercise monitor, send reminders about medication refills, flu shots, and mammograms, and even provide a social networking approach where you can interact with other patients in your physician's practice if you want to.

Case Study: The Blue Button Initiative

The federal government's Blue Button Initiative is like a PHR on steroids. As of August 2012, more than 1 million veterans, military families, and Medicare beneficiaries had downloaded the app, which is now rolling out in the private sector.

The bottom line is that the Blue Button Initiative gets it.

It began in the U.S. Department of Veterans Affairs (VA) with a simple goal, says former VA chief technology officer Peter Levin: to make the entire EHR downloadable for veterans in the quickest possible way.

The first Blue Button version launched in 2010. It was a very simple program, not much more than digitizing personal and health information from the veteran. The app wasn't integrated with the veteran's EHR, but, Levin knew, that was just a matter of time. As soon as you provide patients with any kind of information, he says, the battlements have been breached and the rest of the "castle of medical data" crumbles.

Today, the VA is the only healthcare provider in the United States that makes the entire medical record—"everything we know about the veteran," says Levin—available to the patient.

Users can access demographic information; information about active problems; admission and discharge summaries; progress notes; all lab reports, vitals and readings; and pathology, radiology, and EKG reports. They can also enter data such as their diet and physical activity through integrated journal apps. The app incorporates the VA's continuity of care document, which contains a summary of the individual's essential health and medical care information in a format (XML) that can be accessed regardless of the platform used. The goal is to provide for effective continued

Case Study: The Blue Button Initiative

care and avoid problems with transition of care.

In the United States, such initiatives are supported by federally mandated "meaningful use" requirements designed to move the EHR from just a record-keeping vehicle to one that is used to improve patient care, engagement, and outcomes. The effort is occurring in various stages, with stage 2, implemented in late 2011, requiring that patients be able to not only access their medical information, but transmit and download it. Stage 3 requirements are expected to require that patients be able to enter their own data into their chart.

Private companies and organizations can freely license the Blue Button image and software to develop compatible apps. For instance, Northrop Grumman developed a mobile application that displays Blue Button information on a cellphone, while Humetrix offers a set of mobile applications that allows for the automated access and download of Blue Button records using personal smartphones or USB devices and the direct and secure transfer of these records, by either "push" or "pull," to a healthcare provider's tablet or computer.

To encourage companies to jump on the Blue Button bandwagon by integrating the technology into other mHealth technologies, the Office of the National Coordinator for Health Information Technology instituted the Blue Button Pledge, which has signed on 450 partners that are either data holders or organizations that have the kind of public influence needed to spread the word about the initiative. One goal is to have those organizations use a common format for patient data so it can be accessed across platforms and enable consumers to allow access to their Blue Button data via third-party apps without having to sign in every time or manually download their records. The basic pledge is "to empower individuals to be partners in their health IT."

The goal is to have all health and medical information coming into and leaving from the Blue Button app in an automatic, interoperable manner, says Levin. So prescription refills are sent from the app to the doctor and pharmacy; appointment reminders

> ## Case Study: The Blue Button Initiative
>
> are pushed through the app; lab results appear automatically; sensors that track your heart rate when you run or your blood sugar level if you have diabetes automatically feed the data into the app.
>
> "We're going to provide superior service, improve outcomes, lower costs, and make people glad they saw a doctor," Levin says about Blue Button. "That's what giving them the information does."

Systems are also moving to grant patients real-time access to inpatient data and, in the case of a few large healthcare systems, including the Cleveland Clinic, toward a goal of an "open PHR," which provides patient access to the entire chart, including physician and nursing notes. Why? Because patients want it and like it—and it can improve quality.

"Our vision for the Personal Patient Portal is to allow all patients to easily activate an account and give them the tools they need to be engaged in their care," said Lori K. Posk, M.D., an internist at Cleveland Clinic. "Giving patients access to all their test results and physician notes enables a patient to be informed and actively participate in their care. Creating a culture of transparency utilizing a patient portal will improve the quality and the safety of the health care we deliver."

A paper published in the October 2, 2012, issue of the *Annals of Internal Medicine* reported the outcomes of OpenNotes, a "quasi-experimental study" involving

105 primary care sites in Massachusetts, Pennsylvania, and Washington state, and 13,564 patients who were able to review online the notes the doctors wrote after an office visit.[88]

After a year, 87 percent of patients had opened at least one note. Of the 5,391 patients who opened at least one note and completed the post-intervention survey, 77 percent to 87 percent said the open notes helped them feel more in control of their care. Other findings:

- Sixty percent to 78 percent of those taking medications who opened notes had improved medication adherence.

- Twenty percent to 42 percent shared the note(s) with others.

- Twenty-six percent to 36 percent had privacy concerns.

- One percent to 8 percent said the note caused confusion, worry, or offense.

Nearly all patients wanted continued access to their notes when the study ended, and most said that the availability of open notes would be a "somewhat or very important" factor in choosing a future doctor or health plan.

Although physicians were initially worried that providing access to the notes would disrupt workflow and confuse or worry their patients, none of that happened. Office visits did not take more time, nor did clinicians receive more calls or emails from patients. Instead, many said that the notes strengthened their relationships with patients by enhancing trust, transparency, and communication, and that their patients seemed more "activated or empowered." In fact, the doctors' notes triggered behavioral changes in some patients, such as the patient who said he immediately enrolled in Weight Watchers and began exercising daily after reading the doctor's description of him as "mildly obese."

Between 85 percent and 91 percent of physicians concluded that it was a good idea to make the notes available to patients.

At the Cleveland Clinic, where we provide patient access to physician notes, we've found similar results. Our leadership makes clear that our goal is a completely transparent and open medical record. This reflects our view that patients come first.

We know we're unique, but not for long. And yes, we still hear from colleagues and patients across the country and the world about resistance in the provider community to letting patients "see it all." It's true that there are real issues to resolve through careful discussion, education, and thoughtful implementation. Happily, the open record movement seems to be catching on, which, we believe, has significant benefits for patients and providers.

Developing a Personal Health Record?
5 Things You Need to Know

Marcy Mishiwiec, RN, director of Entity Support Services at San Diego-based Sharp HealthCare, offers the following advice to health plans and healthcare systems as they develop their own PHRs.

- **Make the process inclusive.** That means every department

Developing a Personal Health Record?
5 Things You Need to Know

from legal to clinical to regulatory to information technology, she said. Everyone also needs to be in the same room. "This isn't something that can be done by email." Simple things like automating scheduling took seven departments to work through the issues, she said.

- **Use a performance improvement process such as Lean or Six Sigma.** This ensures consistency throughout the process. It also provides a road map. For instance, she said, "We wouldn't let anyone talk about how the product would look until we had first mapped out our current workflow so we understood who needed to be involved. You have to understand what you're automating before you can automate it."

- **Include physicians on all committees and identify physician champions.** "They are the ones who are going to make or break you. If they roll their eyes when the patient asks about the PHR, you're dead."

- **Prepare for the long haul.** This is not a three-month project, but a "change" project. "The technology is incidental to changing behavior," she said. You also need to account for long-term training and support.

- **Include the patient in the planning.** Sharp conducted focus groups with patients as well as clinicians to identify features that were most important. Don't assume that only younger patients will use the system; about 40 percent of Sharp's users are older than 50, with a significant portion of 80-year-olds using the system, she said.

A Web-based Personal Health Record in Borneo, Malaysia

Personal health records are not limited to developed countries like the United States. Their value is recognized worldwide. In Malaysia, researchers from the Information Science & Technology department at Multimedia University in Melaka are developing a dual cellphone and Web-based PHR for use in the remote parts of the country, such as Borneo.[115]

The goal is to track relevant contextual information for health events such as symptoms, record them in a PHR, and save the context in the PHR. Contextual information is accessed via publicly available information on the Internet. The user would enter a problem or symptom into the cellphone PHR and upload the entry to an account on a Web-based PHR. Then the "context processor agent" uses a database or ontology to search for relevant keywords.

For instance, if the user was in Melaka, Malaysia, and entered "itchy spots," the query would contain the words "air pollution" because itching could be a symptom of an allergy to airborne particulates. The query next goes to the cache agent, which checks to see if similar information has been stored locally, such as other people in that location reporting similar symptoms. Then the query is forwarded to Google and millions of Web pages are searched, with the top 20 results displayed. The information is then organized and stored in a table in the PHR, which notifies the user of the search. For instance, the PHR might provide notice that there is an air pollution warning in the region. The information is then stored in the user's cellphone PHR.

What Do Patients Want From the Personalized Health Record?

An Agency for Healthcare Research and Quality survey of 84 patients and 49 caregivers found that nearly 80 percent of patients and 84 percent of caregivers said they would use a PHR at least monthly.[116] Features they were particularly interested in included:

- Health records organization, including medication reconciliation (91 percent), and information on adverse effects, safety, and medical history conflicts of medications (78.5 percent)

- Access to and exchange of health information (doctor, laboratory, and hospital records) (90 percent)

- Email reminders for preventive tests and regular healthcare routines (84 percent)

- Health directives, including end-of-life care and living wills (79 percent)

- Communications with health plans about claims, eligibility, benefits, and prior authorization (75.8 percent)

- Online calendars and reminders (74 percent)

- Personalized health education (71 percent)

- Access to community services (69 percent)

- Healthcare cost management (57 percent)

If You Build It, They Will Come

The opportunities for mHealth integration in the patient/physician relationship are enormous. As of December 2012, the Pew Internet & American Life Project reported that 87 percent of Americans owned cellphones, about half of those smartphones.[112] That same report found that 42 percent of U.S. cellphone owners ages 18 to 29 use their phone to look up health information, up from 29 percent in 2010.[112]

Obviously, there is still room for growth.

The Pew survey found that while nearly 70 percent said they were tracking their own or a loved one's health data, just one in five was using digital technology to track that data.[117]

Another survey, this one of 99 kidney transplant recipients, found that while 90 percent had mobile phones, only 7 percent knew that such phones could monitor their condition remotely. Still, 79 percent said they would use such a system if it didn't cost them anything.[118]

And another Pew report found that just 19 percent of smartphone users said they had downloaded a health-related app, mainly to track their exercise or monitor their diet.[32] As the author of the report said in an interview, the low consumer adoption is "surprising," given the plethora of apps that are available. In the three years Pew has been asking about health applications, she said, demand has been "essentially flat."

We see this as a direct challenge to you developers out there! We need you to develop more engaging apps that meet users' needs, are easy to use, and integrate into a person's life over the long-term. Now get busy and make it happen!

On the Pharmaceutical Side: Mobile Meds

Nearly half of American adults take at least one prescription drug a day, while one in five take three or more, and one in 10 take five or more.[119] A study from Manhattan Research found that a third of online consumers with chronic conditions and 38 percent of caregivers want online/mobile support to manage their medications.[120]

Enter apps like Lowestmed and GoodRX, which allow you to scan local pharmacies from your GPS-enabled smartphone to find the lowest cost prescription. Or apps from pharmacies themselves, which allow you to access your prescription history, scan the medication package to order refills, and identify pills based on features such as imprint and color.

The pharmaceutical industry has developed its own software to help you manage your health. For example, Merck offers a free iPhone app to help migraine sufferers track their headaches, including when and where they occur, triggers, and severity.

Meanwhile, Boehringer Ingelheim is piloting a digital health management service for people with diabetes that provides personalized health advice and digital coaching with wireless monitoring.

This raises an important point about medically related apps: consumers should know who is behind the app, whether their information will be used for marketing purposes, and, just as with any other source, whether the data is accurate and unbiased.

Improving Adherence

Numerous apps target medication adherence, a major problem throughout the globe. Just half of patients with chronic illnesses adhere to long-term therapy. Such nonadherence increases their risk of poor health outcomes, including potentially life-threatening complications, lower quality of life, and premature death. It also increases costs, adding $177 billion annually in total direct and indirect healthcare costs.[121]

Plus, in a value-based reimbursement system, adherence counts. So developing apps that help patients be more adherent—and let providers know just how adherent their patients are—could have significant benefits.

One product on the market is Memotext, which uses a combination of text message reminders and interactive voice recognition to remind patients to take their medications. Another is AdhereTech, a pill bottle that tracks its contents and wirelessly transmits that data to clinicians, as well as sending reminders and triggers to patients to improve adherence.

With GlowCaps, available at Walgreens and other pharmacies, the bottle cap does the communicating, sending a signal to a small light that flashes when it is time for the patient to take the medication. GlowCaps can also order refills and send a monthly report with incentives to the patient and doctor. Again, it's important to note that pharmaceutical companies typically sponsor such devices.

Studies find such approaches can be quite effective. A Cochrane Review of studies on the ability of text messaging to improve adherence to antiretroviral therapy in patients with HIV found that short, weekly text messages reduced the risk of nonadherence after a year by nearly a third and the risk of virologic failure by 17 percent. Another trial evaluating different intervals and lengths of messages found similar outcomes from weekly text messages of any length. Interestingly, there was no difference in adherence between daily text messages and no messages.[122]

A study funded by Microsoft (which makes the personal health tracking platform HealthVault) and conducted by Johns Hopkins University found the technology increased adherence to glaucoma medication by 16 percent (from 51 percent to 67 percent), while a control group, which received no intervention, showed no improvement.[123]

Other technology in development includes digestible radio chips embedded in medications that transmit adherence data to doctors and drug-containing implants that receive wireless signals to inject the medication at certain times.[124]

Such technologies can lead to significant savings in medication costs and nonadherence-related adverse effects. Thus, insurance companies and Medicare are either reimbursing or considering reimbursing for them. The Economist Unit survey found that 37 percent of insurers in developing countries and 25 percent of those in developed countries are reimbursing for such mHealth approaches.[97]

Case Study: Merck Serono

Switzerland-based Merck Serono is an $8.6 billion global pharmaceutical company that specializes in injectable biologic drugs. Rather than abandon a large portfolio of drugs that had gone off patent, the company turned mobile to reinvigorate them by focusing on adherence, rather than overt sales. As Dan Cowling, vice president and managing director of Merck Serono UK and Ireland, told researchers from PwC, half of all scripts are never filled and half of those are never taken. The company developed a Bluetooth app that tracks all injections and feeds the information to a call center. Miss an injection and within 30 minutes you get a call from a nurse. Since implementing the program, the company gained more than 50 percent of new patients in the areas they cover, grew 38 percent in a static growth hormone market, and reduced its workforce by 20 percent, even though the work volume doubled.[125]

Addressing Counterfeit Drugs

Another important area for mHealth in the pharmaceutical arena is in reducing the amount of counterfeit drugs sold, which is estimated to cost between $75 billion and $200 billion a year and causes significant morbidity and mortality.[97] New technology designed to address this problem comes from French mobile phone company Orange. Patients or providers can text a code number on their medication to a server and instantaneously receive a message as to whether that batch is real or fake. The system is being tested in Kenya but still needs financial backing.

Improving Fitness and Chronic Disease with Mobile Health

The explosion of chronic disease in this country—nearly half of Americans have one or more chronic medical conditions such as diabetes, obesity and heart disease—is a major drive of mHealth, says Michael Roizen, M.D., who chairs the Cleveland Clinic's Wellness Institute. "There are two major facts that lead to the inescapable conclusion that we must reach people outside of a medical environment," he said. The first is escalating medical costs that will either lead to rationing or lack of care, and the second is the poor lifestyle choices many Americans make, including poor nutrition, large portion sizes, lack of physical activity and stress management, and tobacco exposure.

Such toxic exposures, he says, contribute to 70 percent of the incidence and prevalence of chronic disease in this country. "Thus, the only way for us to control medical costs is to decrease the influx of chronic disease; and the only way to do that is to reach populations before they get chronic disease or, outside of the medical environment, reverse existing disease."

Which is why you can barely turn around today without bumping into some kind of health and fitness app. An abundance of apps claim to help you lose weight, track your workouts, and assess your sleep patterns. In mid-2012, there were more than 13,000 consumer health apps in the Apple iTunes store, with about 70 percent targeting consumer wellness and fitness (Figure 4-2).[126] But just how well do they work?

Figure 4-2. Health-Related Apps

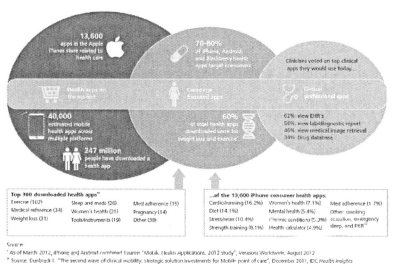

Source: Deloitte. mHealth in an mWorld: How Mobile Technology Is Transforming Health Care. 2012.

A study published in 2012 in *The American Journal of Preventive Medicine* found that overweight adults (N=210) who monitored their diet intake with a personal digital assistant (PDA) that provided daily personalized feedback were more adherent and lost more weight than those who simply tracked their diet via a PDA or paper diary.[127]

Another study evaluated the effect of a mobile phone app that provided patient coaching, as well as a secure messaging center for patient-provider communication and a PHR with additional diabetes information, learning library, and logbook. Providers had access to analyzed patient data linked to standards of care and evidence-based guidelines. Patients entered diabetes-related data into the app and received personalized messages based on the data. They also received an electronic action plan every two-and-a-half months to support their self-management and serve as "previsit" summaries for office visits.

Patients in the intervention group demonstrated a nearly 2 percent decline in their A1C levels compared to 0.7 percent in the usual care group over 12 months regardless of their starting level. That's a huge improvement in a year and extremely clinically relevant.

One problem with all these apps? Consumers download them and then forget them. They're not "sticky" like your bank. They simply don't keep patients actively involved or offer enough value for us to return to them again and again. So they fail. As Eleanor Chye, Ph.D., executive director, Mobility Product, mHealth & Pharma at AT&T, said in an interview: the focus must shift from capturing data to empowering patients to "do something with it."[128]

That's exactly what the Cleveland Clinic is doing with the Enforcer eCoaching program Dr. Roizen developed. The premise is simple: participants email their "coach" daily updates about their physical activity, nutritional patterns, smoking cessation efforts, etc., and receive personalized responses back that encourage positive behavior and gently suggest changes in not-so-positive behaviors. So far, there are six-month programs targeting diabetes, hypertension, weight loss and smoking cessation.

The results, he says, are tremendous. In a soon-to-be-published study, he reports that the average weight loss in the e-coaching group over 26 weeks, while the smoking cessation group had an 84 percent success rate in quitting and remaining smoking free.

The program is one that everyone in the healthcare system could be using within the next five to 10 years, he says, and one that he envisions integrating with the EHR to drive preventive care in the clinical setting.

The e-coaching works, says Dr. Roizen, because it provides an intrinsic reward to participants through the positive feedback from the coach. As the participant begins to see real progress, that, in and of itself, becomes the reward.

Creating the Perfect App

If we were to design the perfect app, whether for healthcare providers or consumers, it would be:

- Secure and private
- Interactive
- Intuitive to use
- Portable across platforms
- Integrated into the EHR and PHR
- Able to transmit data wirelessly
- Built from the user perspective, not the developer perspective
- Tested with its intended audience
- Designed to meet a personal need
- Designed to become part of your personal ecosystem, like Facebook

> ## Way Cool: Tictrac
>
> It's not just doctors who have problems managing the vast amounts of data mHealth devices and applications generate; pity the poor consumer with 45 apps on her phone, all collecting bits of data about her emotional and physical well-being.
>
> Enter Tictrac, an app that integrates with different third-party services like RunKeeper, Fitbit, Withings, Google Calendar, Gmail, Foursquare, Facebook, Twitter, Last.fm, and more to track everything from food consumption and mood to spending. It then runs the information through an algorithm and spits the results back at you in the form of a unified dashboard of well-being so you can better understand yourself—and your life.

The Virtual Office Visit

So, will mHealth eliminate the face-to-face office visit? Will we even *need* doctors if we can train computers to do what they do? Of course we will!

"Digital health technology in any form is not meant (or should not be meant, at least) to be a complete substitution for human input or interaction," said Harrisonburg, Pennsylvania-based digital health technology consultant David Lee Scher, M.D., in an interview. "Most times the digital tech will be an adjunct by adding either computerized algorithmic suggestions, a face without the hand holding, an anonymous source adding the comfort of privacy, or a sense of self-management. Many times the digital interaction will prompt a face-to-face, one that is more meaningful than the routine visit or follow-up just to review test results. This type of visit will be prompted by patient-derived significant data transmission or a concern on the part of the provider prompted by an actionable alert. It does not serve either patients or providers to view technology as either a substitute or threat."

Nonetheless, virtual visits are here to stay. WellPoint, Inc., the second-largest insurer in the United States, is now paying for video visits in all its plans, providing software that allows consumers to interact with their doctors on demand using their laptops or video-enabled smartphones or tablets. Other insurers offer the option for certain employer groups, many of which are including remote consults as part of their benefits. Mercer Consulting estimates that 15 percent of the largest employers are using some form of telemedicine, while another 39 percent are considering it.[129]

The main reason? Cost savings. One study on the use of virtual mental health sessions among 98,609 VA patients, most of whom were 45 or older, found it reduced psychiatric hospital admissions by 24 percent and decreased the average time spent in the hospital by 26 percent.[50]

Plus, patients *like* telehealth visits. A Spanish study in which HIV-infected patients received traditional face-to-face visits for one year, and then email and webcam visits for a year, found that 85 percent of patients said they were happy with the virtual visits. This approach to visits reduced the amount of time doctors spent with patients and eliminated scheduling problems while still being both pleasing and effective.[49]

Text Messaging—The New Doctor?

About 80 percent of cellphone users use their phones to send or receive text messages, or short message service (SMS). More than 90 percent are between ages 18 and 49. However, just 9 percent of adults in the United States receive health-related texts, representing a tremendous opportunity in the mHealth world.[117]

We'll highlight how SMS is being used in the developing world in Chapter 6, but in the meantime, here are some outcomes from SMS programs in the United States.

- Simply sending three text messages for three weeks to diabetes patients led to dramatically improved adherence to medication, as well as increased healthy behaviors and improved understanding of their disease.[130]

- The first published randomized evaluation of the text4baby program, a government-sponsored initiative that delivers text messages to underserved pregnant women and new mothers to help them change their health and healthcare beliefs, practices, and behaviors found the program works and leads to improved clinical outcomes. The study assigned 123 women to receive the intervention or regular care. It found that women receiving text4baby messages felt nearly three times as ready to be a new mother as those who weren't and were less likely to say they would drink alcohol during pregnancy.[131] Longer-term evaluations are under way.

- A study of 31 women with bulimia evaluated the effects of 12 weekly group cognitive behavioral therapy sessions along with a text messaging protocol. The women texted each night about how many binge eating and purging episodes they'd had that day, and they rated their urges to binge and purge. Their responses triggered an automated message tailored to their symptoms. Nearly 90 percent of the women adhered to the program, demonstrating significant improvements in their depression, eating disorder, and night eating.[132]

- An Australian study sent eight messages about sexual health or sun safety over three months to subscribers to an advertising site. Those who received the sexual health messages had significantly higher sexual health knowledge and fewer sexual partners than those who only received messages about sun safety, while those who received the sun safety messages were significantly more likely to wear a hat than those who received only the sexual health messages.[133] (We admit we are disappointed they didn't ask about wearing hats during sex.)

Other text-based or mobile phone-related approaches show significant benefits in the areas of teen depression prevention, HIV testing, improved sexual health, increased physical activity, and healthy eating, and even attendance in primary care clinics.[134-136] Text-based messaging can also reduce health disparities across racial and demographic groups.[137]

One study evaluated the key components for a successful text messaging health promotion program:[138]

- Informal language

- Positive, relevant, short messages

- Funny or rhymed messages

- Messages that tied into particular annual events

Case Study: Telemedicine and the Veterans Administration[139]

The U.S. Department of Veterans Affairs (VA) set out in 2010 to completely transform the way its beneficiaries interacted with the healthcare system. That involved, among other initiatives, creating patient-centered medical homes in all primary care practices and, as part of that, instituting the Care Coordination/Home Telehealth (CCHT) program.

They program telehealth services to veterans in local clinics or their homes using an integrated, Web-based portal that contains information the veteran enters, self-management tools, integration with the EHR, health education materials, and secure messaging with healthcare providers.

To date, more than 500,000 veterans have used the telehealth program to do everything from measuring their blood pressure and heart rate and transmit the results to their physicians to holding virtual "office" visits with specialists. The system can even be used for minor acute illnesses like the flu. A nurse conducts a virtual basic assessment using a specialized video camera pointed in the patient's ears, nose, and throat.

The Elderly and mHealth

The coming tsunami of elderly in the United States (thank you Baby Boomers!) provides numerous opportunities for mHealth. What, you say? Older people don't want to use computers and other digital technology.

You couldn't be more wrong.

A survey of nearly 3,000 U.S. adults 65 and older found that more than half were ready to use the Internet to manage their health and communicate with their physicians, while a report from the Pew Internet & American Life Project published in mid-2012 found that, for the first time, half of adults in this age range are online.[32]

Nearly all of those surveyed used a computer to look up health information, with just 10 percent using a tablet. About half of *those* used their tablet for healthcare management. This demographic, however, is less likely than younger adults to download health management apps. One reason could be that just 11 percent own smartphones.[140]

But they're pretty comfortable communicating via computer. A study (conducted between 1998 and 2003) evaluating email communication between patients ages 65 to 79 and their primary care physicians found that while few patients communicated this way with their doctors, about half would like to, with African Americans and Hispanics more interested than whites.[141]

It's time to ditch these old stereotypes.

mHealth for Families and Loved Ones

It's not just patients who can benefit from mHealth. Families and loved ones who act as caregivers also benefit. The U.S. Department of Veterans Affairs (VA) recognized this when it started a pilot program in 2013 to provide iPads preloaded with a variety of healthcare apps to more than 1,000 families who receive benefits to care for severely wounded veterans.

The tablets feature a suite of integrated apps to track everything from pain levels in the injured veteran to a journaling program for the caregiver (one of the most requested apps from caregivers) that allows them to log all activities and share the information with the healthcare team. There are apps that let the veteran assign surrogacy functions to the caregiver, that integrate all appointments into a calendar, and that provide information on medication. One app, PTSD Coach, which provides post-traumatic stress disorder screening and symptom tracking, is programmed to alert the patient's primary care provider if scores suggest high symptoms.

The VA will assess the effectiveness of the program by comparing the healthcare burden and utilization between families who receive the iPad and those who don't.

One key to success? Physician enthusiasm and communication skills. Patients whose doctors were excited about using email were 1.3 times more likely to also be excited, while patients who already thought their doctors were good communicators were 1.6 times more likely to be enthusiastic than those who rated their physician's communication skills as just "fair" or "good."

Can They Handle It?

A review of 68 studies on mHealth and telemedicine for people 60 and older found that most patients using the technology were living at home and able to handle the devices by themselves. Most of the interventions were monitoring, such as measuring vital signs, but also included personal interactions with the provider through video conferencing or telephone. The authors concluded that the studies showed "predominantly positive results" with a clear trend toward better results for behavioral endpoints such as medication or diet adherence and self-efficacy.[142]

There is a more important role for mHealth in the elderly population: helping older people maintain their independence and providing peace of mind to caregivers.

For instance, GeriJoy is a talking virtual dog developed at the Massachusetts Institute of Technology that is designed to monitor people with dementia and improve their interpersonal connections.

GeriJoy runs on any tablet. Caregivers put the tablet on display in a room where the elderly person spends a lot of time. The "dog" can talk with the person, calm them down, orient them to the time of day and scheduled activities, and report on their status to caregivers. The sound is streamed over the Internet to a live GeriJoy representative who can alert the caregiver to any problems. Family can also share photos and other events with the person by uploading them to a family portal website. The "dog" uses this content to engage patients in conversations, helping reinforce family memories and relationships.

Other systems, such as the LivingWell@Home program, provide sensors, telehealth, and personal emergency response services for the elderly. LivingWell@Home is currently being evaluated in a clinical study involving 1,600 people throughout five states.

The Power of Play: Games as Game Changes

More healthcare apps that target consumers integrate our innate desire for fun and competition into the software. Yes, we're talking games. The growth in the gamification of mHealth was clear during the 2012 mHealth Alliance meeting in Washington, D.C., where gaming garnered its own pavilion in the exhibit arena.

Venture capitalists are touting gamification as one of the hottest mobile technology trends (and putting their money where their predictions are); businesses are turning to games to retain customers, train employees, and increase revenue; and, of course, developers are turning to games to change behavior.

Stamford, Conn., research firm Gartner, Inc., estimates that by 2015, more than half of organizations that manage innovation processes will gamify those processes.[143]

"Gamification is about applying game-design thinking to non-game applications to make them more fun and engaging. Tap into people's natural desire to compete and play, and it results in high levels of engagement."

Adam Swann
Gamification Comes of Age.
Forbes. July 16, 2012.

A game in the healthcare domain is not really about winning or losing, says Michael Fergusson, CEO of game developer Ayogo ("ayo" is another word for mancala, the oldest board game in the world; "go" refers to the Asian strategy game, one of the most sophisticated games in the world).

"We like to say that our business is the application of the behavioral psychology of games to health care to help people with chronic diseases manage their condition more effectively," he said. In other words, using a game to change.

The Robert Wood Johnson Foundation sees significance of games in health care. It is funding the Games for Health Initiative, which brings together a multidisciplinary team of experts, including disease management specialists, to identify how evidence-based approaches to chronic disease management can be turned into games.

An important component of games for health is incorporating a social network, Fergusson said. Studies already find that social networks influence behavior. For instance, recently published studies support the idea that obesity can spread (or not spread) through social ties.[144]

The interactivity of games linked to social networks also drives behaviors that people might not display in a static game, he said. For instance, would you ever annoy your Facebook friends by putting ads on their walls? Most people would say no. Until they play Farmville and send pleas for "money" to buy sheep and rose bushes.

The popularity of Farmville, Fergusson said, is driven not by the game itself, but by the opportunity to interact with other players and with one's social network.

Ayogo used this understanding when it teamed with the Joslin Diabetes Center and the Diabetes Hands Foundation, with financial support from Boehringer Ingelheim Pharmaceuticals, to develop HealthSeeker, a Facebook game for kids with diabetes or at risk of developing the disease. Users pick lifestyle goals they'd like to achieve, then choose from various "missions" to help them reach their goals. Each mission contains activities players can incorporate into their daily lives. When players complete a mission, they move up a level and collect points. With points, they earn badges and can move to even higher levels. The game is designed to be played with Facebook friends so the players provide support and feedback, as well as competition.

Another Ayogo-developed diabetes application works apart from Facebook but still has the same social network philosophy. Diabesties (as in "best friend"), created in conjunction with the College Diabetes Network, is designed to help teens with type 1 diabetes during the often-difficult transition to college. It teams students with others on campus who have type 1 diabetes so they can share things like blood glucose ratings and nutritional tips through texts and instant messaging. "We create a reciprocal social obligation between the students," Fergusson said, in which each wants to do better than the other.

The most important thing about Diabesties isn't that the student sends her results to another student; it's that she's receiving another student's results, triggering the competitiveness that is part of every well-designed game.

Another advantage to social games is that they provide constant feedback on progress, increasing a sense of self-efficacy, Fergusson said. The competition motivates players to "step up their game" and play harder and longer to reach their goals because it provides bragging rights to their social networks. Also critically important, social networks provide a "space," such as the wall in Facebook, to provide and receive support, encouragement, and feedback.

Techniques that turn an app into a game include:

- Giving points that lead to rewards such as badges

- Moving up levels

- Displaying leaderboards

- Using virtual currency

- Competing against other virtual players

- Providing the ability to trade, give away, or sell points

- Offering real-time feedback

Games also activate the brain's reward circuitry, triggering dopamine release in the same way any pleasurable activity does. This creates a feedback loop (feels good—you want to do it more— you do it again—you get another burst of dopamine) that encourages more frequent play. If the incentives and rewards within the game are tied to health-related behaviors, then the feedback loop is rewarding those behaviors in a short-term manner rather than the long-term reward of "better health down the road" that we know rarely motivates patients.

One challenge with health-related games is making money. "Taking care of health is work," Fergusson said. "We don't want to pay for applications like that." The answer lies in convincing insurance companies and employers to pay for it. Another possibility is that as more clinicians are reimbursed based on value rather than volume, they will pay for it since they have a financial incentive to ensure a healthier population.

Will Patients Pay for mHealth?

There is a lot of skepticism over the question of whether consumers will shell out money for health-related mHealth apps and devices. The experts who insist that they won't should review the results of a consumer survey from the Health Research Institute. The company estimates the consumer market for these devices between $7.7 billion and $43 billion, based on how much consumers say they will pay out-of-pocket.[145] Here's what the consumers told them:

- Forty percent said they would pay for remote monitoring devices and apps and a monthly service fee to send data automatically to their doctors, although they want to pay less than $10 for the app and less than $75 for the device.

Will Patients Pay for mHealth?

- Those who delayed care more than five times in the last year are more willing to pay out-of-pocket for doctor visits, electronic or in-person.

- Only half of consumers surveyed said they would buy mobile technology for their health. Of those, a fifth said they would use it to monitor fitness or well-being, while a fifth wanted their doctors to monitor their health via the technology.

- Consumers who are in good health are more likely to pay for apps than those in poor health.

A final example to consider in closing Chapter 4 is on GeoPalz and their Zambee device.

Mobile Health and Mobile Incentives

What if our health status could be turned into a kind of "health currency" in which you garner credits via your mobile phone for healthy behaviors, like exercising, reporting your blood glucose level, and taking your medication? That's just what some developers are offering with their apps. GeoPalz, for instance, is a pedometer for kids. Parents create an online account for their kids, who earn "points" they can spend on sports equipment and video game systems by logging their steps. The points can even be used to purchase items on Amazon.

Zamzee, a small device that connects to a gamified website, also measures physical activity in kids, rewarding them with points they can redeem for prizes like gift cards, donations to causes, iPods, and more.

A six-month study on Zamzee that involved 448 middle-school–aged youth, half of whom received just the device and half of whom also had access to the motivational website, found that those using both increased their moderate-to-vigorous physical activity by 59 percent overall, with girls increasing it by 102 percent. The results were presented at the 2012 Obesity Society's

Mobile Health and Mobile Incentives

Annual Scientific Meeting in San Antonio, Texas.

Those who used the device consistently also demonstrated improved blood sugar levels, reducing their risk of diabetes. Explaining the success of the device and game, Steve Cole, Ph.D., vice president of research and development at HopeLab, which developed the app, and professor of medicine at the University of California, Los Angeles, said in an interview, "We worked very hard to eradicate education from this. For instance, there were no references to health or the word 'exercise' because kids just don't want to hear such talk." Like any good game, Zamzee relied on intrinsic motivation to change behavior.[146]

Talk about motivation to get moving!

Chapter 4: Key Takeaways

✓ Consumerization is a powerful driver in the development and adoption of mHealth. Soon, mHealth will not be a nice-to-have, but a must-have in healthcare delivery.

✓ Consumers are ready to incorporate mHealth into their interactions with the healthcare system and to use it to improve and maintain their own health.

✓ Consumers probably have the fewest barriers to using mHealth among all the players. At this stage they aren't even as worried about privacy as we might think.

✓ mHealth is a critical component of patient engagement and patient-centered care.

✓ mHealth applications must be fun, interactive, simple to use, and able to retain the patient over the long term (stickiness).

✓ The gamification of mHealth is growing in size and importance as an opportunity to engage patients and improve health.

✓ Virtual "office visits" are no longer a thing of the future but are occurring today in all areas of health care.

Chapter 5. mHealth: Its Role in a Value-based Reimbursement Model

"Widespread adoption [of mHealth] is dependent on the reimbursement model. If these new devices are not covered by insurance, it's unlikely patients will purchase these technologies out-of-pocket, especially safety-net populations."

NEHI
Getting to Value: Eleven Chronic Disease Technologies to Watch. June 2012

If you have health insurance through Aetna, one of the largest health insurers in the United States, then you might have an app on your mobile phone that enables you to find a local doctor, view your personal health record, learn about your coverage and benefits, integrate with your GPS to locate the nearest urgent care center (with turn-by-turn directions), and even use your phone as your identification card.

Yet, just three years ago Aetna had little-to-no mobile capacity, said Dan Brostek, who heads the company's department of member and consumer engagement. Today, Aetna has invested more than $1 billion in health management and health IT solutions, spending some of that money to purchase Healthagen, the parent company of iTriage, a leading mobile health company with one of the most frequently downloaded (and used) apps in the world.

In the past two years, Aetna also launched its CarePass platform, which enables consumers to seamlessly integrate data from a plethora of health and wellness apps into one location. To stimulate further development, the company opened a developer portal to encourage the creation of other health and fitness apps that integrate with CarePass and has awarded grants up to $100,000 to app developers.

"The intent is to allow consumers at large or Aetna members to leverage and interact with their top health apps and then have that data be aggregated within the CarePass environment," Brostek said. The system "goes beyond a personal health record," he said, because it's not just a repository for data but a way to make that data active and turn the experience into a goal-oriented approach designed to improve health and increase engagement.

Way Cool: Bike Your Way Through France—Virtually

Aetna is also building its own apps, like the Passage app it developed in collaboration with Microsoft for the Windows 8 platform. The app is designed to transform the classic workout routine from one spent watching CNN or listening to music to one that transports the user to exotic locations like London and Paris via real-time pictures in Instagram, restaurant reviews through Yelp, and insider travel tips and facts about the locations as people progress through the virtual route.

To encourage wellness among its members, Aetna lets all members and employees download the premium version of the Mindbloom Life game for free. The app uses behavioral science, personalized rich media, and social gaming techniques to help users identify what's most important in their lives and what drives them, and to take meaningful action in those areas, which include health.

The goal, Aetna says, is to "empower consumers by putting their health in their own hands, resulting in healthcare delivery that is more convenient, connected, and cost-effective."

But the dive into mHealth has other benefits for Aetna, benefits that align perfectly with the goals of healthcare reform: drive savings, encourage patient engagement, and improve outcomes.

That's why Aetna is far from the only payer integrating mHealth into its services as a way to control costs.

UnitedHealthcare, which covers more than 14 million people around the country, offers its Health4Me app. It lets members check claims and account balances, locate nearby urgent care facilities and emergency rooms (ERs), and access a registered nurse 24 hours per day, seven days per week for advice regarding any kind of medical question.

Have a question for customer service? Forget navigating phone trees and sitting on hold. Just select the type of question you have from within the app and someone calls you back on your mobile.

One unique offering from UnitedHealthcare—one we think could be transformative in a system desperate for cost transparency—is its myHealthcare Cost Estimator, which gives users the ability to comparison shop for more than 100 services based on cost and quality in nearly 50 markets. It even creates side-by-side quality comparisons for treatments at specific facilities.

The estimates, which are personalized to reflect the user's own health plan benefits, are based on actual contracted rates with physicians, hospitals, clinics, and other healthcare providers. The tool also builds "care paths," showing users what they should expect throughout the course of treatment. Quality and cost information is directly connected to in-network hospitals and physicians, and alternate treatment options are provided so consumers can have an "informed conversation" with their physician.

Key features of the program include:

- Cost estimates for more than 47 geographic areas covering more than 100 treatments and procedures, such as surgeries, lab tests, radiology tests, and office visits. The estimates are personalized for the user, identifying all out-of-pocket costs, costs employers will pay, and real-time account balances available in eligible health savings accounts that can be used to pay out-of-pocket costs,

- Quality and cost information for 240,000 physicians and hospitals,

- Presentation of common alternate treatment options to educate patients on their choices,

- Educational information about how the benefits work and how costs are determined.

UnitedHealthCare also provides a medication and disease management application that enables patients to manage their care using two-way text messaging on their mobile phones. Called CareSpeak, patients can report not only their medication intake to clinicians, but also biometric data such as blood glucose levels, blood pressure, and weight. They receive educational and motivational messages, as well as incentives and rewards for meeting their health goals.

WellPoint, which covers 36 million people, teamed with Verizon Wireless for a pilot program involving 100 WellPoint members with chronic diseases. Members received a smartphone and were assigned a health coach they could contact any time, day or night, by phone or face-to-face videoconferencing.[147]

Case Study: AT&T and mHealth

In 2011, AT&T, one of the largest self-insured employers in the country, initiated a pilot program with its Health Care Services Corporation, the largest consumer-owned health plan in the country with more than 13 million members, to see if the FDA-approved DiabetesManager app could impact patient management of diabetes. The company chose DiabetesManager, which was developed by AT&T partner WellDoc, based on the results of a randomized clinical trial that showed its use reduced hemoglobin A1C levels (a measure of good diabetes control) by 1.6 percent in the user group versus 0.7 percent in the control group.

The 156 users in the six-month pilot received instant feedback and coaching based on real-time data, while their healthcare providers received historical reports and analysis, all within an infrastructure compliant with the federal Health Insurance Portability and Accountability Act, or HIPAA.

After six months, 88 percent of users rated DiabetesManager as a "highly useful" tool to help them manage their diabetes, 78 percent said they would continue to use the tool after the initial pilot period, and 93 percent said they would recommend the tool to someone else.

In addition, the pilot resulted in far higher customer "stickiness"

Case Study: AT&T and mHealth

than most apps, which 74 percent of users abandon after the first 10 uses. In the DiabetesManager pilot, nearly two-thirds of users entered the program at least once a week at least two out of every four weeks, while a third used it at least once a week in at least three out of every four weeks. At the end of the six-month pilot, 45 percent were still using it compared to 10 percent of users for all mobile applications.[148]

Similar pilots with healthcare companies Centene and Alere yielded similar results.

Why the big jump by payers into mHealth? One word: cost. Just take a look at Table 1 and you get a clear picture of the potential of mHealth to rein in costs and utilization, particularly in today's primarily fee-for-service model. The potential will be even larger as the United States and other countries move toward value-based reimbursement models. For instance:

- A remote patient monitoring system from the U.S. Department of Veterans Affairs (VA) called Care Coordination/Home Telehealth slashed inpatient days by 40 percent. The program cost $1,600 per patient per year, while the VA's typical home-based program of nurse visits costs $13,121 per patient per year. Between 2004 and 2007, the program reduced the use of healthcare services for patients with diabetes by more than 20 percent; for patients with hypertension by 30 percent; and for patients with congestive heart failure by 26 percent.[149] The VHA estimates that half its patient population could be cared for with home telemedicine technologies.[150]

- Remote, postsurgical pulse oximetry monitoring at Dartmouth-Hitchcock Medical Center in New Hampshire saved an estimated $1.4 million on one floor alone by reducing complications, rescue events, transfers to the intensive care unit, lengths of stay, and readmissions.[109]

- Partners HealthCare in Boston used a telemonitoring and education program called Connected Cardiac Care for patients with congestive heart failure and realized a 50 percent drop in heart failure–related readmissions and 44 percent drop in non-heart failure readmissions among the 1,200 patients enrolled in the program. The savings were impressive: more than $10 million since 2006, or about $8,000 per patient even after deducting the cost of the program. Just as impressive? Patients better understood their condition and learned new self-management skills, while the program also resulted in high levels of clinician and patient acceptability and satisfaction.[149]

- Centura Health, the largest integrated healthcare provider in Colorado, combined its clinical call center and remote monitoring telehealth program to try and reduce 30-day readmission rates for patients with heart failure, chronic obstructive pulmonary disease (COPD), and diabetes by 2 percent. They met that goal and then some, reducing rates in the three areas by a whopping 62 percent, emergency department visits by 92 percent, and home visit frequency from an average of two or three a week to an average of three over a 60-day period.[149]

Table 5-1. Cost Utilization Savings from mHealth

	Where	What	Result
Diabetes	Pennsylvania	Post-discharge remote monitoring	42% drop in overall cost per patient
	Cleveland	Cellphone size wireless transmitter transfers vital signs to electronic health record	71% increase in number of days between office visits
Congestive heart failure	Trans-European-Network-Home-Care Management System	Remote monitoring of patients who received implantable cardiac defibrillators	35% drop in inpatient length of stay; 10% reduction in office visits; 65% drop in home health visits
Chronic obstructive pulmonary disease	Canada	Remote monitoring of patients with severe respiratory illness	Reduced hospital admissions by 50%; acute home exacerbations by 55%; hospital costs by 17%

Source: PwC Health Research Institute. *Healthcare Unwired*, 2010. Available at: http://www.mobilemarketer.com/cms/lib/9599.pdf

Another reason payers can't afford to *not* integrate mHealth into their services is the potential of mHealth to reduce administrative expenses. Always a topic of interest to payers, this became even more important in 2010 with the implementation of the Affordable Care Act (ACA). The ACA requires that insurers spend no more than 15 percent or 20 percent (depending on the insurer) of the premium dollar on non-healthcare related expenses, such as administrative expenses. If they go over, they have to refund the money to the customer. Digitizing services provided by high-cost employees enables the same kind of virtual, cost-saving services that banks and airlines have been providing for years.

Going mobile can also increase reimbursement for payers, says Ram Davaloor, COO and founder of El Segundo, Calif., based iSpaceGlobal, an information technology company. His company has developed a mobile platform that pings physicians if they enter the wrong diagnosis code. In a world of value-based, not fee-for-service, reimbursement, the diagnosis code takes on greater importance than procedure-related codes because it is the diagnosis code that drives risk-adjusted reimbursement. His company has also helped insurers turn their paper-based, people-heavy health risk assessments into apps, saving one company nearly $2 million.

Meanwhile, an enrollment app for Medicare Advantage that the company developed is saving on administrative costs and getting member information into the computer system within hours versus the five days or more the paper-based system required.

Finally, the ability of mHealth to better engage patients in their own health care and improve shared decision-making has cost savings potential, as well.

Any initiatives that can bring down costs while maintaining or improving quality are critical in today's market in which employers refuse to tolerate any more double-digit premium hikes like those in years past and are demanding better returns on their premium investments.

Plus, after 2014, large premium hikes in the individual market may be vetted by state insurance boards—something few health plans want to experience. Interestingly, though, a PwC survey found that the individually insured are most likely to use apps to monitor their health and to pay out of pocket for electronic physician visits, remote monitoring devices and services, and monthly fees for mHealth apps, likely because they tend to have higher out-of-pocket costs.[151]

However, as Figure 5-1 shows, payer reimbursement for mHealth in the United States still lags behind that of developing countries. One reason for the slow movement here? The third-party payer system, which limits the role of consumers in paying for medical services. "Public and private health insurers are primarily responsible for paying for healthcare," notes a PwC report, "and they generally have not pushed for adoption."[151] Other challenges include licensing regulations, reimbursement policies, and scalability of the evidence to show that the benefits of pilot programs will apply to large-scale population health.[151]

Figure 5-1. mHealth Services and Payers

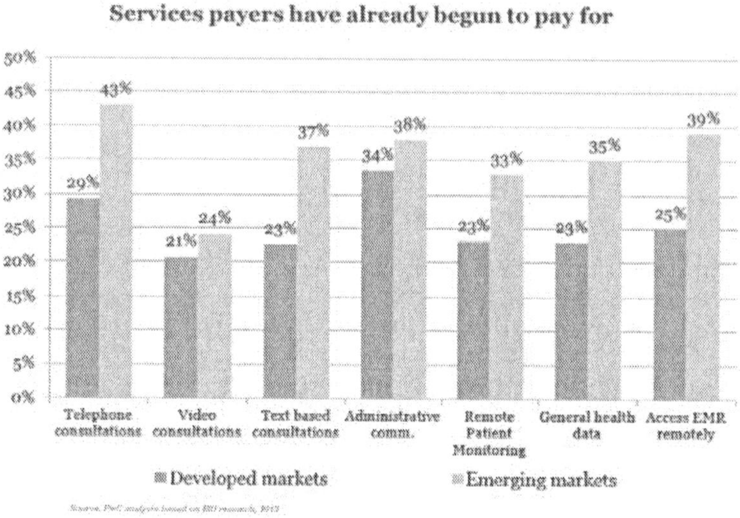

Services payers have already begun to pay for

Source, PwC analysis based on BMI research, 2012

iTriage: 8.5 Million Downloads and Counting

It's a simple idea. Type your symptoms into an app, press a button, and voila! Possible diagnoses. Not only that, but you can use the app to make doctor appointments, store your personal health record, save medication refill reminders, and learn about thousands of medications, diseases, and procedures. You can even use it to find out wait times if you need an ambulance and, in certain markets, preregister at an urgent care center or emergency room.

That simple idea, called iTriage, is now one of the top five health and medical apps downloaded by iPhone and Android users, with one of the longest retention rates in the industry. The app, available in 80 countries, is used about 3.5 million times a month, and its users have posted nearly 1 million reviews in the app marketplaces, most of them four or five stars. "People make decisions based on the information we give them," said Wayne Guerra, M.D., the company's chief medical officer.

iTriage: 8.5 Million Downloads and Counting

The company also listens to its customers, reading every one of the reviews it receives each day (to date, that totals 750,000). "That's how we get our features," said cofounder and CEO Peter Hudson, M.D. For instance, users asked for a medication database and refill reminder, which iTriage added, including an allergy app to track allergies. "It's built for people who take charge of their health," he said.

iTriage's parent company, Healthagen, has been recognized by the White House as an example of innovation, growth, and impact on the healthcare industry, and as a leader in effective health care industry change. In fact, its CEO was Michele Obama's guest at the 2013 State of the Union address. In 2011, Aetna purchased the company for an undisclosed amount. Not bad for a 4-year-old company started by two emergency room physicians.

iTriage is also built to help payers reduce costs by directing patients to urgent care centers instead of emergency departments for conditions like a sprained ankle. That's why health insurers and accountable care organizations (ACOs) include iTriage as part of their consumer engagement solutions. The company can customize the app for the member's insurance plan, providing reminders on reducing costs, lists of in-network providers, and links to their personal health record. The app even tells users if they have a telehealth benefit and how to use it.

It's not just patients that are using it. Check the cellphone or tablet of many clinicians and you'll find the app. "They use it to keep track of the thousands of conditions and medications out there," Dr. Guerra said.

In addition, Healthagen partners with more than 600 hospital systems to provide institution-specific information and, in many areas, allow patients to register at the emergency room or urgent care center before they arrive and check waiting times. It is also part of a "technology stack" that Aetna is selling to ACOs and other healthcare entities. The stack includes three

iTriage: 8.5 Million Downloads and Counting

components from Aetna subsidiaries: a health information exchange from Medicity; a care management and rules engine from Active CareTeam that provides clinical decision support services and a desktop-based workflow tool to track, monitor, coordinate, and report on patient health outcomes; and, of course, iTriage.

Arizona-based Banner Health, which runs a Medicare Pioneer ACO, was one of the first companies to purchase the stack. The app is designed to recommend a doctor within the ACO, if appropriate, and direct patients to lower-cost alternatives like physical therapy for back pain to, hopefully, avoid surgery.

The purchase makes sense under the ACO reimbursement model. If Banner meets certain quality and cost goals, it is eligible to share in any cost savings. Aetna was so certain of the value of its program that it is sharing the risk for those savings with Banner and will be paid for the technology only if the health system can generate demonstrable savings.

Payers Turn to Telemedicine to Reduce Costs

Telemedicine: "The delivery of health care services, where distance is a critical factor, by all health care professionals using information and communications technologies for the exchange of valid information for diagnosis, treatment and prevention of disease and injuries, research and evaluation, and for the continuing education of health care providers, all in the interests of advancing the health of individuals and their communities."[152]

World Health Organization

For the biggest cost savings from the mobile world, payers are going beyond apps to the world of telemedicine, also called "telehealth." A 2012 Towers Watson survey of 72 large employers representing 1.7 million employees found that while just 8 percent currently offered telehealth services, nearly a third (28 percent) planned to offer it within 12 months.[153]

Here's what's happening on the payer side:

- Virginia-based health insurer Coventry Health Care provides its members with telephone and video access to a local physician 24 hours a day, seven days a week, via the mobile health and telemedicine company CareClix.

- Blue Cross and Blue Shield (BCBS) of North Carolina, the technology company American Well, and Walgreens teamed up in 2012 to provide telehealth services to thousands of BCBS employees throughout the state. The system lets employees receive healthcare consultations from nurse practitioners, health coaches, or nutritionists through two-way video, secure text chat, or phone.

Aetna recently changed its payment policy to allow payment for certain telemedicine codes for Level III NCQA Patient-Centered Medical Home physicians. The goal is to increase physician accessibility and accentuate the "patient-centered nature of high-quality care." Aetna is also placing health kiosks in the offices of large employers so employees can conduct their own basic self-assessments and receive reports on their weight, blood pressure, temperature, and blood oxygen level. They can print the results to give to their physicians or send them directly into their personal health record. They can also receive personalized care through a live, on-demand voice or video consultation with a state-licensed, board-certified doctor. The video consultation costs $35 or less.

- WellPoint members can hold online video consultations with contracted physicians 24/7 in some states as part of a "Web walk-in" program (the company plans to expand the service for smartphones and tablets later in 2013). A major goal of the program is to reduce spending on emergency department services by providing increased access to clinicians.[154] In 2013, WellPoint added video consults from on-call specialists, with payment claim automatically submitted.

- Cigna will begin offering MDlive service to its self-insured customers in 2014. The service allows members to request online video, phone, or email consultations with primary care physicians for nonurgent issues. Doctors are available 24/7 and respond within an average of 11 minutes. Members can even access the service from the insurer's mobile app.

Telehealth can reduce mortality rates, as well as initial hospital admissions and emergency department visits.[150]

So, do these initiatives save money? You bet.

A 2013 article in *Health Affairs* found that an online clinic run by HealthPartners Health Plan in Minneapolis delivered savings of $88 per care episode—plus a 98 percent patient satisfaction rating—for simple, acute medical conditions.[155] The program, called virtuwell currently offered in Minnesota, Wisconsin, and

Michigan, is available around the clock and provides treatment for 40 simple medical conditions.

Patients complete an online interview and nurses or physician assistants review the data, make the diagnosis, and, within about half an hour, email or text the treatment plan. If needed, they send a prescription electronically to a pharmacy. In addition, patients or caregivers can initiate a phone call at any time during the process.

Between 2010 and 2012, more than 40,000 people received treatment plans through the service. About 56,000 others whose symptoms exceeded the scope of practice were referred to other providers. The most common diagnoses were sinusitis, urinary tract infection (UTI), conjunctivitis, and upper respiratory infection.

About 85 percent of those using the service were covered by insurance, with the fee for the visit $40 or less, depending on the contract with the insurance company. The service is also the first in the nation to be authorized for Medicare services.

Not only were the users satisfied, but, anecdotally at least, HealthPartners physicians were too, in part because they helped design and run the program.

While the virtuwell visits cost, on average, $88 less than an office visit, that amount varied by condition and setting. For instance, for acute sinusitis, conjunctivitis, and UTIs, the virtuwell treatment cost $20 to $30 less than "walk-in" clinics like those in drugstores; $80 to $142 less than office visits; $82 to $124 less than urgent care visits; and $159 to $469 less than emergency department visits.

Even more impressive is the fact that 89 percent to 95 percent of the virtuwell visits for those three conditions were resolved with the online visit and did not require a face-to-face visit, a rate comparable to those of patients treated in a walk-in clinic. In addition, about 90 percent of the virtuwell visits were *instead of*, not in addition to, office visits, with patients saying that if the service were not available, they would have seen someone face-to-face. This supports the idea that the service did not increase demand by encouraging patients who might otherwise have waited to see if the situation resolved at home to seek care.

Another interesting finding? In keeping with national guidelines, virtuwell providers were far less likely to prescribe antibiotics for acute bronchitis than providers who saw patients in person. As the study authors wrote: "[This] suggests that a well-designed online venue can provide appropriate care. Additionally, it may suggest that the online venue better supports providers trying to use antibiotics appropriately or that patients inclined to push clinicians for antibiotics may be less successful in doing so when treated online."

The program has benefits for large employers beyond simple cost savings, the authors also noted, because it could significantly reduce the absenteeism that occurs when employees have to miss work to see a healthcare provider.

"Virtuwell's early results suggest that online care has the potential to meet the 'Triple Aim' goals of a better health care experience for patients, improved population health, and more affordable health care—especially for conditions typically associated with primary care."

Courneya PT, Palattao KJ, Gallagher JM. HealthPartners' Online Clinic for Simple Conditions Delivers Savings of $88 Per Episode and High Patient Approval. *Health Aff (Millwood)*. 2013;32(2):385-392.

Aetna is also taking telemedicine and its potential quite seriously. "Traditionally, 'laying of hands' has been required in order for a provider to be paid for the delivery of health services," said Dan Brostek, Aetna's head of head of member and consumer engagement, which is why insurers have typically not paid for telephone calls and emails. No doubt the lack of payment has greatly limited adoption of remote visits by providers.

But, he said, with advances in telemedicine such as mobile devices and two-way videoconferencing, the visits have become much more like "in-person" visits. "We believe telemedicine can play a critical role in improving health and managing chronic disease, while increasing member satisfaction," he said. The cost savings will come from reducing nonmedically necessary emergency department visits and other after-hours care.

Aetna began supporting telemedicine in 2006 with its RelayHealth program, which reimburses participating primary care physicians and more than 30 specialists for online consultations and Web-based visits with Aetna patients who have nonurgent health concerns. Patients can only use the system for certain conditions and only with their established doctors, which, Brostek said, helps preserve the continuity of care and the doctor-patient relationship.

"This is care that members may not seek otherwise due to time and access constraints," Brostek said. Overcoming that barrier is particularly important today when most patients have chronic conditions that would benefit from ongoing care to prevent acute (and more expensive) exacerbations. "Telemedicine solutions remove the barriers because they are available after hours, on the weekends, or even during lunch breaks from almost anywhere," he said.

Adoption of these options is strong, Brostek said. And yet, he stressed,

> "We have always been clear that we don't see telemedicine options as an alternative to the establishment and maintenance of patient care delivered by primary care physicians. Rather, we see that telemedicine may complement the patient-physician relationship by making it easier for physicians to deliver care effectively and efficiently, facilitate communication with patients, and help improve patient safety."

Aetna is also working to leverage the information collected during telemedicine visits with applications such as Medicity, ActiveHealth, and iNexx so the information can be securely shared with the member's primary care provider. He calls it a "game changer" that can improve primary care provider and patient engagement and partnership. "Telemedicine with integrated health information technology support can work to improve the healthcare system," he said.

The telemedicine trend isn't limited to health insurers. A *Wall Street Journal* article published in late 2012 noted that many large companies, including Home Depot Inc., Booz & Company, and Westinghouse Electric Co., are moving to include remote consults in their benefits. And the California Public Employees' Retirement System started testing a service that offers phone and online visits from Teladoc to 350,000 enrollees.[129]

Way Cool: Watson

Scientists at IBM are developing the next generation of Watson supercomputer (yes, the one that beat a human in *Jeopardy*) to improve medical care. The technology can extract relevant clinical information from unstructured data such as medical notes, discharge summaries, registration forms, etc., to provide the kind of analytics that could improve outcomes. One way cool component? A button to submit treatment suggestions to the health insurer to receive near-instant approval and dramatically reduce the administrative headaches many now experience.

The reason is simple: cost. Not only can telemedicine reduce direct medical costs, but it can slash indirect medical costs by reducing absenteeism and presenteeism (when an employee is physically present but not productive). The Integrated Benefits Institute estimates that health-related poor productivity costs employers about $227 billion a year.[156]

Teledoc: The Newest Employee Benefit

One of the newest employee benefits is 24/7 access to a physician or other healthcare provider through services like Teladoc. The Dallas-based company, which bills itself as the first and largest provider of telehealth medical consults in the United States, has more than 4.5 individual members, with most receiving the benefit through their employer.

Even middle-sized firms like Colin Konschak's company, Divurgent, with just under 100 employees, offer the service. Divurgent is a management-consulting firm with employees throughout the United States who travel every week of the year. This makes Teladoc an incredibly convenient—and important—benefit.

"It's more efficient," said human resources director Marydawn Bovatsek. "You don't have to take off from work or have your child miss school." For instance, when her son had a reaction to an antibiotic after normal office hours, she considered taking him to the emergency room. Instead, she called Teladoc, spoke to a U.S.-based, board-certified physician, described the symptoms, and received a recommendation to take him to his primary care physician the next day.

The benefit costs $10 a month for family coverage and is linked to employee health insurance and online medical records so the physician can access information while on the call or video conference.

Another reason for the interest? Telemedicine has significant potential to reduce costly readmissions, which occur in one in five patients and represent nearly a fifth of overall Medicare spending.[99] Beginning in 2012, Medicare began penalizing hospitals 1 percent of the reimbursement for readmissions within 30 days in patients with heart failure, pneumonia, and acute myocardial infarction. A report from NEHI (formerly the New England Health institute) found a 60 percent reduction in hospital readmissions compared to standard care and a 50 percent reduction compared to disease management programs that don't use remote monitoring. The authors concluded that remote patient monitoring could prevent between 460,000 and 627,000 heart failure-related readmissions each year, saving the healthcare system (primarily Medicare) up to $6.4 billion a year.[150]

Figure 5-2 shows the readmission rate reductions that two large health plans realized through the technology.

You can read more about the use of telemedicine and mHealth in reducing readmissions in Chapter 3, and about mHealth on the global stage in Chapter 6.

Some companies and healthcare systems are considering making these systems revenue generators by selling subscriptions to families after the first 30 days of post-discharge monitoring. It would cost families far less than another hospitalization, not to mention providing peace of mind and, possibly, reducing visits to providers.[157]

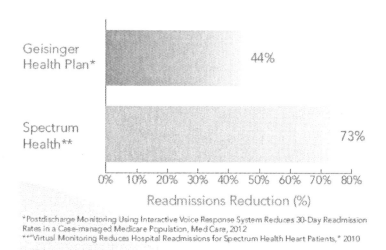

Figure 5-2. Using Telehealth to Reduce Readmissions

Geisinger Health Plan* — 44%

Spectrum Health** — 73%

Readmissions Reduction (%)

*Postdischarge Monitoring Using Interactive Voice Response System Reduces 30-Day Readmission Rates in a Case-managed Medicare Population, MedCare, 2012
**"Virtual Monitoring Reduces Hospital Readmissions for Spectrum Health Heart Patients," 2010

Source: Qualcomm Life, Inc. Delivering Accountable Care with Remote Monitoring for Chronic Disease Management. 2012. Available at: http://www.qualcommlife.com/

Way Cool: Using Kinect to Save Money

Researchers found that using something as simple as Microsoft's Kinect gaming system, an Azure connection to create virtual networks, and an Office 365 account at a total cost of about $500 could replace or augment existing telemedicine systems that cost $25,000 or more. They estimated the system could save the U.S. healthcare system more than $30 billion a year because patients wouldn't need to be transported from rural areas to specialty hospitals. This could also lower the risk of infection.[158]

Barriers to Widespread Adoption of Telehealth

"The present and potential uses of telemedicine are constrained by overlapping and often inconsistent and inadequate regulatory frameworks and technical standards imposed by governments and professional medical organizations."

Gupta A, Sao D.

The Constitutionality of Current Legal Barriers to Telemedicine in the United States: Analysis and Future Directions of Its Relationship to National and International Health Care Reform. *Health Matrix.* 2011;21.

There are numerous barriers to the widespread adoption of telehealth, including lack of financial and clinical outcomes data and reimbursement for the approach. Few of the smaller fee-for-service plans cover telehealth services unless patients live in rural areas.[150] However, changing reimbursement structures such as bundling and capitation may be one way to overcome this barrier. Something has to be done, particularly at the public payer level. A PwC report found that less than half of Medicaid and Medicare patients said they would pay out-of-pocket for electronic doctor visits.[151]

Another barrier is the electronic health record. If you don't have one, then telehealth is pretty limited. Even if you do have one, integrating it with the telehealth system can be challenging. (Hint: If you're buying a new EHR system make sure it's telehealth ready.)[150]

We believe that the adoption and impact of telehealth will increase when you can add, review, and update health information in one place. So, at the Cleveland Clinic we place a high premium on concepts like the EHR as the "single source of truth" and decision support that is embedded in the user's workflow. It is also why we recently announced that, in an effort to promote transparency and sharing within the EHR, we will be applying the same open records policy we have had for our paper charts to the EHR and related patient portal, providing patients with *everything* in their medical charts, including physician notes. We are also actively working on new technologies that make it easier for patients to enter their own information.

A significant challenge lies in state and federal laws related to the physician/patient relationship. Most states require face-to-face interactions before clinicians can prescribe medications or require that an in-state physician supervise nurse practitioners and physician assistants. In addition, only a handful of states permit out-of-state licensed physicians to consult with patients whether in person or virtually.

Meanwhile, outdated federal reimbursement policies limit the use of telemedicine under Medicare and other federal health coverage programs.

The federal government may finally be getting its act together when it comes to telehealth with the Telehealth Promotion Act of 2012 (H.R. 6719). The act, which as of spring 2013 was gaining steam in Congress, would establish a federal reimbursement policy wherein "no [medical] benefit covered shall be excluded solely because it is furnished via a telecommunications system." If passed, the bill would increase access to telemedicine within Medicare, Medicaid, the Children's Health Insurance Program (CHIP), TRICARE, federal employee health plans, and the Department of Veterans Affairs. The bill also allows providers licensed at the state level to treat patients remotely anywhere in the nation (for these insurance programs).

Other changes in the bill that apply to federal programs include:

- Incentivizing hospitals to lower readmissions with telemedicine by offering them a share of the total cost savings.

- Exempting ACOs from telehealth fee-for-service restrictions and allowing them to use telemedicine as an equivalent substitute for in-person care.

- Adjusting reimbursement timelines for home health to better facilitate remote patient monitoring.

- Creating a telemedicine service option in Medicaid to treat high-risk pregnancies.

These changes are great (if the bill passes), but they don't cover those with commercial insurance. That's where state policy changes are needed. These should include not only changes in licensing requirements, but mandates for insurance coverage of telehealth. To date, just 15 states have laws requiring that health plans cover and reimburse for telemedicine, with just four (California, Pennsylvania, Texas, and Vermont) extending that mandate to Medicaid programs.

However, 44 states cover some form of telehealth in their Medicaid programs. (Connecticut, Iowa, Massachusetts, New Hampshire, New Jersey, Rhode Island, and the District of Columbia do not reimburse for any telehealth under their Medicaid programs.)

Those 44 states all reimburse for live video, although some only pay for it when provided in underserved areas. Only seven offer some reimbursement for asynchronous telehealth (the electronic transmission of medical information, such as digital images, documents, and prerecorded videos, between medical professionals). Just 10 states reimburse for remote patient monitoring, and just three Medicaid programs reimburse for all three forms of telehealth.[159] Most do not allow prescribing without a face-to-face visit.

The good news is that in early 2013, 13 states were considering some form of telehealth legislation, with six states and the District of Columbia introducing bills that cover its use in private insurance.

"The technology of telehealth is well ahead of the socialization of the telehealth idea and we are at a tipping point for utilization to begin taking off."

David Jacobson,
WellPoint's Staff Vice President of Business Development, State Sponsored Business,
quoted in *Healthcare Unwired*, PwC Health Research Institute, 2010

Better Prescribing, Lower Costs

Doctors often prescribe medication without considering the patient's health insurance, says Jeff Yaniga, vice president of Los Angeles-based DRX, which provides Web-based comparison tools, technology, and data. That drives up costs for both patients and health plans. But what if health plans gave their members a tool to empower them to learn more about their

Better Prescribing, Lower Costs

prescriptions?

That's just what DRX has developed. The company's DrugCompare suite of apps tells patients if the drug is covered by their insurance, how much it costs, what pharmacy provides the best price, and if there are other drugs in the same class that could provide the same benefits but at a lower cost. The beauty of the app? Members can use it right in the doctor's office before the doctor writes the prescription.

A company analysis of user activity in 2011 found it saved users (including health plans) an estimated $1.3 billion. Had all users acted on the information they received, savings would have been closer to $12 billion.

Chapter 5: Key Takeaways

✓ We expect payers and employers to embrace mHealth, particularly telehealth, as an important tool in their arsenal to improve quality and reduce costs.

✓ We have to confront and overcome barriers to the integration of mHealth with reimbursement.

✓ We need to decide how to reimburse for mHealth-related activities, including who pays for the initial investment in equipment for services like telemedicine.

✓ We need changes at the state and federal level to encourage telehealth and to provide fair reimbursement for its use, as well as changes to state licensing laws for physicians and nurses so they can treat patients in any state and prescribe medications without face-to-face visits.

✓ We need to find a way to integrate apps and other mHealth services that payers provide with the patient's personal health record and find a way to mine the information that comes in through these apps to personalize the patient's health care, improve quality, and reduce costs.

Chapter 6. mHealth on the Global Stage

"Of the 3 billion people who live on less than the equivalent of $2 per day, 1 billion have no access to the healthcare system ... Yet, in the midst of so little infrastructure, leapfrog innovations to serve the poor abound."

Advancing the Dialogue on Mobile Finance and Mobile Health. mHealth Alliance. Washington DC, 2012.

Text messages to improve maternal and child health. Mobile phones equipped with electrocardiogram technology. Lensless microscopes that "diagnose" HIV and malaria using only a mobile phone. Research, data collection, and training accomplished virtually, through a cellphone in some of the most remote, poorest regions of the world, where just a single doctor is often caring for thousands of people.

This is not the stuff of fantasy. This is real, and it is happening in Bangladesh, Tanzania, Kenya—throughout Africa—as well as Central and South America, the Mideast, and elsewhere. Places with no power, no landlines, and few hospitals. And it's working.

You need only to read the program for the December 2012 mHealth Summit in Washington, D.C. For the first time, conference organizers included the first global health track.

Attendees packed panels with titles like: "The Road Ahead: The Future of Mobile Technologies for Global Health," "Using Mobiles to Improve Maternal & Newborn Health," and "Scale-Up: Creating an Enabling Environment." Panelists came from throughout the world, including Nepal, Brazil, Tanzania, Peshawar, Uganda, and the World Health Organization (WHO).

The reason for the interest is easy to understand once you look at the numbers. Although healthcare spending throughout the world exceeds $4.2 trillion, nearly 90 percent of it is consumed by 20 industrialized countries that contain just 16 percent of the population. The United States alone, with 5 percent of the population, spends nearly half. The rest of the world shares 11 percent of health spending, but suffers from nearly *95 percent of the diseases.*[116]

The state of health care in developing countries? "It's an appalling situation," said Alain B. Labrique, Ph.D., director of the Johns Hopkins University Global mHealth Initiative in Baltimore. "The challenges are tremendous."

MHealth could change all that as a 2013 PriceWaterhouseCoopers (PwC) report entitled, *Connected Life. The Impact of the Connected Life Over the Next Five Years*, illustrated, that literally hundreds of thousands of lives will be saved across the African continent just through the continued implementation and adoption of mHealth technologies.

In addition, consider the findings of a PwC survey of residents in 10 developed and underdeveloped countries (Figure 6-1):[97]

- Sixty-one percent of those surveyed in the developing world were aware of the term "mobile health" versus 37 percent in developed markets.

- Fifty-nine percent of those surveyed in the developing world use at least one mHealth application or service versus 35 percent in the developed world.

- More doctors in developing countries offer mHealth services than doctors in developed countries.

Figure 6-1. Emerging Market Patients' Expectations of mHealth

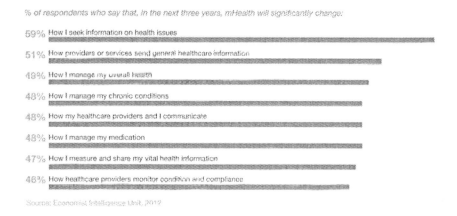

% of respondents who say that, in the next three years, mHealth will significantly change:

59% How I seek information on health issues

51% How providers or services send general healthcare information

49% How I manage my overall health

48% How I manage my chronic conditions

48% How my healthcare providers and I communicate

48% How I manage my medication

47% How I measure and share my vital health information

46% How healthcare providers monitor condition and compliance

Source: Economist Intelligence Unit, 2012

Source: PwC analysis based on Economist Intelligence Unit research, 2012.

How is it possible that mHealth is more entrenched and more understood in poor, underdeveloped countries than in rich countries like the United States? In a word: need.

Unlike much of the developed world, people in developing countries are orphaned from their own healthcare systems. Many live 100 miles or more from the nearest hospital and most lack transportation. There are few doctors. For these people, mHealth isn't a luxury. It's a necessity. It's the only way to access modern medical care.

In addition to the greater need and demand, the governments of some developing countries are not as hampered by entrenched interests (also known as lobbyists and politicians) as governments in the developed world. Thus, they can develop an mHealth-based healthcare system more quickly and with fewer administrative hurdles than the West.[97]

This is possible even though people in these countries often don't have running water, paved roads, reliable electricity, or landlines. It's possible because they *do* have the one piece of technology that makes mHealth possible: a mobile phone.[160] The United Nation's International Telecommunication Union estimates that nearly 80 percent of people in the developing world have a mobile phone subscription, with 62 percent of Internet users living in underdeveloped countries.[161] Even people who don't own phones have access to one through family and friends.

In developing countries, the mobile phone is a leapfrog technology since, given infrastructure limitations, they never fully adopted personal computers. Instead, they went right from analog communication to mobile phones, making the phones their own portable "computer."

While there are 11 hospital beds and 305 computers for every 5,000 people in the developing world, there are 2,293 mobile phones.[162] By the end of 2011, 105 countries sported more mobile-cellular subscriptions than people, including Botswana, Gabon, and South Africa.[31] Overall, an estimated 76 percent of the world's 6 billion cellphone subscriptions are in developing countries.

Farmers use their phones to learn the latest crop prices; people without bank accounts use them to send money to relatives; teachers in African villages use them to contact parents about their children's whereabouts. In Ghana, cab drivers use phones equipped with special sensors to test and report air pollution levels. And throughout the developing world, activists use text messages and other social media to help organize protests.[139] Just consider the Arab Spring of 2011.

Then consider Malawi, a small African country with a population of 16 million. Just one in 63 residents owns a landline, but one in five owns a cellphone. It's similar in Tanzania, where just 12 percent of the population has a bank account, but more than half have mobile phone subscriptions.[115] Of all developing regions, sub-Saharan Africa has the fastest mobile growth rate in the world. In 2000, just 1 percent of residents there owned a mobile phone. By 2012, that percentage had jumped to 54 percent.[146]

Figure 6-2 depicts mobile subscribers for 10 other countries.

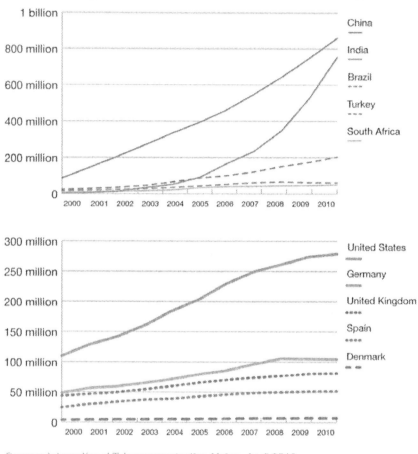

Figure 6-2. Mobile Subscribers for 10 Countries

Source: International Telecommunication Union, April 2012

What a change from a decade ago, when Dr. Labrique and his team worked on a project in Bangladesh at two sites about 18 miles apart. Communication was so difficult, he said, that "we were looking into investing in carrier pigeons because there was no way to make a landline call."

By 2009, however, that had radically changed. "We had faster broadband Internet in rural Bangladesh than we had in Baltimore."

Cellphones as Lifelines

Cellphones are increasingly serving as lifelines that connect isolated people to the care they need, making possible tasks once unthinkable in the poorest regions of the world, said Dr. Labrique. Among them:

- **Collecting data.** "There is nothing more powerful in global health than the ability to count," he said. "If you can't quantify the problem, you can't argue for political and financial support." Enabling community health workers to send data via their mobiles directly into a database simplifies and improves data collection, reduces errors, and improves work satisfaction for staff who now don't have to carry heavy bags full of paper. Most importantly, it enables national health systems to track and monitor basic health indicators at every level and make decisions accordingly. The mobile phone literally creates a digital web for these communities.

- **Training**. Most medical care in developing countries is provided not by physicians, but by trained community health workers. Simply being able to text a question about medication dosage to a physician hundreds of miles away improves care. Mobile devices can also be preloaded with dosage calculators, clinical guidelines, decision-making protocols, medication facts, and other important pieces of information that a health worker might not be able to remember.[117]

- **Diagnosing**. Healthcare workers can now send photos and other pieces of clinical information to physicians or nurses hundreds of miles away, enabling the physician to quickly diagnose a patient and recommend the appropriate treatment.

- **Preventing and treating disease**. Reminders, interactive games, and other tools are being used to encourage residents to seek medical help when needed, undergo important testing, and get vaccines and other medicines.

- **Disaster response.** Cellphones can be used to determine water safety, locate survivors, and triage the injured after earthquakes, floods, and other natural disasters. As Dan Diamond, M.D., a member of Medical Teams International told an mHIMSS reporter: the smartphone is one of his most important medical tools. Dr. Diamond uses the phone for a variety of tasks, one of the most important of which is quickly searching medical references for information about diseases, infections, medications, and injuries he hasn't seen before. The phone's GPS also helps track supplies and medical personnel, find the injured, and reroute supply vehicles when roads are impassable. Its barcode scanning can help track inventory, while social media apps are invaluable in communicating with a diverse population of disaster specialists and residents in the disaster zone.[128]

Case Study: Starting from Scratch in Abu Dhabi

Why would the Cleveland Clinic build a $1.6 billion, 360-bed, 2,500-employee hospital complex in Abu Dhabi, a small country of the United Arab Emirates (UAE), where just 600,000 people live in its largest city? Because we can. And because it's needed. And because it offers a unique opportunity to partner with the UAE to design and build the hospital of tomorrow and create what we expect will be a global healthcare destination.

The hospital, which should open in late 2014, will be owned by the Abu Dhabi government and Mubadala Development Co, PJSC, although we will operate it. Other fun facts:

- Nearly 3 billion people are within a six-hour flight of the hospital.

- It can be expanded to 490 beds.

- It will employ about 170 physicians and 1,500 nurses and allied health professionals.

- Physicians must meet the same standards we require of those at the U.S. Cleveland Clinic, including being North American board-certified (or equivalent).

- It will include more than 30 medical and surgical specialties.

- It will include four royal suites.

- It is the largest structural steel building in the UAE, weighing more than 30,000 tons.

Our goal is to bring the underlying philosophy of the Cleveland Clinic to the UAE, particularly our patient-centric, group-model focus.

"The vision from the beginning was to create a digital hospital—a smart building," said Michael Reagin, chief information officer for Cleveland Clinic Abu Dhabi and the project's first employee. Along those lines, the hospital will open with a Stage 6 Electronic Medical Record Adoption Model from the first day, something just 9.1 percent of U.S. hospitals had achieved by the end of first

Case Study: Starting from Scratch in Abu Dhabi

quarter 2013.[163]

Building a digital hospital means creating an interoperable, converged network, with all building systems, security, entertainment, mobility, and biomedical services existing on one common infrastructure. "This has never been done," said Reagan. Of course, losing connectivity means you can't even turn the lights on, so the system has a highly redundant infrastructure.

Building such a hospital is even more impressive when you consider that the landscape of health care and infrastructure in Abu Dhabi is about 20 years behind that of the United States, he said, with advanced telecommunications still in its infancy. "We almost needed a waiver from the government to install a 10 gigabyte network," Reagan said, which is common practice at the Cleveland Clinic. The country doesn't even have a fiber-optic infrastructure yet, although that is beginning to change. "It still feels like the 1980s and 1990s did in the U.S. from a network perspective," Reagan said.

When it comes to mobility, the hospital started with cellphones, not computers. Most people in the country—from the highest executive to taxi drivers and day laborers—carry at least two cellphones at all times, Reagan said, and even professionals rarely have home computers. "It's amazing how connected people are 24/7 on their mobile phones," he said. For instance, when he tried to give an in-person presentation about the hospital, he received a lukewarm reception. But once he provided the presentation via mobile phone, "it was a completely different conversation."

"Texting is the way they communicate," he said. "Everything is done that way," from withdrawing money from the bank to making a dinner reservation to arranging a delivery. No one, he says, uses voice mail.

Texting, or short message service (SMS), is also already entrenched in the healthcare system, he said. Healthcare providers send patients SMS reminders for appointments and driving directions, among other services. They don't provide access to medical records or online scheduling via mobile like healthcare entities in the United States.

"Such portals are not widely accepted here," said Reagan. However, the hospital will go live with the EPIC MyChart personal health record system within 90 days of seeing the first patients, he said, as a way to enable communication between patients and providers.

They will start small, initially offering only "culturally appropriate" information online and then adding services as they move forward. All built, of course, on the mobile phone platform.

One advantage to the technological focus is that people in the UAE equate high tech with high quality and will make purchasing decisions (including purchasing health care) based on the technology profile of the company, Reagan said.

On the clinical side, "there's a wide desire to use technology such as telemedicine and home monitoring to reduce costs and provide value," he said, particularly as the hospital wrestles with the question of how to provide the best care for people who would otherwise have to travel hours to reach the hospital.

In the past three years, Reagan and his team have learned several valuable lessons about building a state-of-the-art hospital and attendant healthcare system from scratch:

- **Understand the infrastructure.** While the telecommunications infrastructure in Abu Dhabi has improved in just the three years Reagan has been there, "it continues to be challenging." They must try to identify the challenges and design a flexible, dynamic system that can overcome those barriers today and be tweaked to address future challenges.

- **Understand the culture.** In the UAE, customer service is king. "The decision to visit a facility or doctor is influenced by the service you get there," he said, even more so than patient perception of the quality of care. That includes things like valet parking, room service for patients, and

Case Study: Starting from Scratch in Abu Dhabi

regular offerings of coffee and tea, all of which are built into the hospital's operations. It is also important that any new services the hospital implements work the first time out—no beta testing. "Word of mouth rules everything," Reagan said, even which healthcare provider people choose. "If someone has a good or bad experience, word travels very fast." People are also very mobile in the UAE, he said, commuting across countries for work. The digital network must operate on all available platforms, not just the one in the UAE.

- **Assess the regulatory climate.** The new hospital will use the most recent billing standards and reimbursement approaches, including ICD-10 (still to be adopted in the United States) and diagnosis-related payment group (DRG) systems. However, that requires moving very rapidly from a nonelectric, non-connected billing system to one that is very dependent on connectivity, he said. "That's a big transformation that has consumed a lot of time and energy."

- **Understand differences in medical practice.** For instance, things U.S. physicians take for granted, like being able to prescribe medications electronically, are unknown in the UAE.

- **Start recruiting early.** Finding and recruiting talented information technology (IT) professionals in a part of the world that is experiencing double-digit growth in IT has been a challenge, he said.

And the biggest lesson for other organizations looking to launch similar projects from scratch? "Design the system around mobile and smartphones."

Table 6-1. Health Care in the United States vs. the United Arab Emirates

Healthcare Parameter	United States	United Arab Emirates
Maternal mortality rate	21 deaths/100,000 live births	12 deaths/100,000 live births
Infant mortality rate	5.9 deaths/1,000 live births	11.25 deaths/1,000 live births
Life expectancy at birth	78.62	76.91
Health expenditures	17.9 percent of GDP	3.7 percent of GDP
Physician density	2.7 physicians/1,000 population	1.9 physicians/1,000 population
Hospital bed density	3 beds/1,000 population	1.9 beds/1,000 population

Source: The World Factbook. Central Intelligence Agency. 2013.

Arming Community Healthcare Workers With mHealth

Community health workers are often the first and only point of care for most of the "bottom billion" and the world's rural poor.

Isolation and lack of training limit their ability to provide little more than basic care, often separate from the larger healthcare system. mHealth has the potential to change that. "Mobile systems now exist to address gaps which, until recently, seemed intractable," says Dr. Labrique. Such systems can provide continued skills development and training to frontline health workers, integrating them as full-fledged members of their health systems.[164]

A good example is Malawi's St. Gabriel's Hospital in Namitete. The hospital serves 250,000 people spread over a 100-mile radius. To reach people in the surrounding villages, it relies on 600 volunteer community health workers, many of whom do not have access to motorized transport.

These workers are the hospital's eyes and ears. They travel on foot among the rural communities to confirm that villagers take their medication as directed, remind them about medical appointments, deliver test results, offer advice, field questions, and fill out detailed health records. Until recently, all that recordkeeping was done on paper, requiring that they walk dozens of miles from villages to the hospital to submit reports. Because it took so long to walk from place to place, the hospital received just 25 reports a month.

Then the hospital gave 75 workers cellphones at a total cost of $250. Armed with the phones, the workers could text hospital staff to:

- Tell them when patients need refills on their medication so the hospital's nurse could bring them on her next regular visit.

- Update them when patients die so the nurse doesn't waste a trip to deliver morphine and other palliative care.

- Report on whether patients are taking medicines correctly, particularly important when treating HIV- and tuberculosis (TB)-infected individuals, when missing doses could result in treatment-resistant disease.

- Relay patient questions to a physician or nurse and receive an immediate reply.

- Request emergency care.

- Ask for more supplies.

- Make sure they understand the purpose and dosage of the medications they deliver to patients.

The results were startling. The hospital saved $2,750 in six months, mainly in fuel costs because the nurse and TB coordinator didn't waste gas by driving from village to village. Since workers no longer had to walk long distances to and from the hospital, they could care for more patients. Filed reports jumped from 25 a month when hand-delivered to 400 a month via text. In just six months, the hospital doubled the number of TB patients under its care.[165]

For a similar initiative, the Uganda Health Information Network armed healthcare workers with smartphones. The workers use them to input health information about everything from medication usage to disease incidence to supply stocks. The data is emailed over a cellular network to a server in another city, which then routes the message and information to the right people who send back messages and information (if needed). Educational content is also sent to the workers several times a week. The net cost savings: 25 percent in the first six months, mostly because the devices eliminated the need to travel. Health workers also reported increased job satisfaction since a mobile phone is a lot easier to carry than 10 pounds of paper reports.[162,166]

"Over the past five years, hundreds of pilot projects across the globe have tested mHealth strategies to increase the capacity of community health workers and improve the quality of care received by the populations they serve.... These systems enable tasks that were previously thought to be logistically impossible—enumeration of

populations; registration of pregnancies, births and deaths; scheduling of antenatal, postpartum, and immunization visits with accountability for missed or delayed contacts; and providing at least a rudimentary health record. Importantly, these systems also provide a means to improve system efficiencies, from worker management to monitoring supply chains (including identifying counterfeit medications), as well as real-time monitoring and reporting of vital events and system performance.

"Most importantly, the most vital function of mobile phones, often lost in the whirlwind of innovation—voice communication—is a central facet of the mHealth revolution, allowing workers to access peer and supervisor guidance when and where they need it."

Alain B. Labrique, Ph.D.,
Director, Johns Hopkins University Global mHealth Initiative

mHealth in the Developing World: Maternal and Child Health

The WHO estimates that 99 percent of the 800 women who die during pregnancy or childbirth every day live in developing countries.[167] And, although infant mortality rates have improved in recent years, they are still dismal in these parts of the world, especially in sub-Saharan Africa, where a newborn is more likely to die within its first month of life than one born anywhere else in the world. Overall, a child born in Africa is six times more likely to die before its first birthday than one born in Europe or other parts of the developed world.[118]

Yet, up to 75 percent of maternal deaths and 70 percent of newborn deaths are preventable.[168]

Fixing this problem seems like an impossible task. In many developing countries, huge distances separate pregnant women from the health professionals who could care for them—and those health professionals are few and far between. For instance, there is just one doctor for every 100,000 Malawians. Indeed, the Malawian doctor shortage is so severe that more Malawian physicians work in Manchester, England, than in their country of birth.[165]

So, it's no surprise that Malawi has a maternal mortality rate of 460 per 100,000 women (the United States rate is 21 per 100,000), and a neonatal death rate of 79 per 1,000 live births, compared to the U.S. rate of six out of 1,000.[169]

This is, however, an area where mHealth can—and is—making a difference. In fact, a review of 34 articles published in *Maternal Child Health Journal* found that mHealth helps just by minimizing the time it takes for a mother or infant to receive urgent care.[168]

Malawi participates in the VillageReach program, which provides a free maternal, newborn, and child health hotline and mobile tips and reminders. Between 2011 and 2012, the hotline received about 500 calls a month. Seventy-seven percent of users reported changing behaviors around pregnancy and childbirth, such as maternal nutrition and complementary feeding, and more than 70 percent said they learned something new from the messages.[170]

In Bangladesh, where maternal mortality is the leading cause of death among women, more than 90 percent of births occur outside of a hospital, and neonatal deaths comprise more than half (57 percent) of fatalities under the age of 5. The Telenor Group, a mobile communication company, launched a Mobiles4Health initiative to teach pregnant women how to care for themselves and alert them to early warning signs of infant problems. It also provides family planning and breastfeeding advice. The program launched in 2011, with a goal of reaching 500,000 women by 2014.[171]

Another program in Bangladesh has women trained to text healthcare workers or midwives when their labor starts so the healthcare workers can assist in the delivery. Since the program launched, 89 percent of women enrolled had assisted births. The project was so successful that researchers at Johns Hopkins University expanded it to enable easier scheduling of prenatal care visits, as well as post-childbirth health checks.[131] Pregnant women there can also get a reduced rate on their cell service if they register their cellphone numbers to allow them to receive free prenatal advice targeted for their gestation age. The program has not yet been evaluated for success.

And in south Asia, where a quarter of all infants are born prematurely, health officials often don't hear about the infant until a day or two after the birth, which is the highest risk time for mortality, says Dr. Labrique. With a cellphone, the mother can text a healthcare worker that she's in labor, "and we can deploy skilled health workers to the home to be there either as part of the care team or to facilitate referrals when a crisis occurs," he said. "This opens up a whole new paradigm of public health strategy that we didn't have access to before."

A major maternal/child health initiative in the developing world is the Mobile Alliance for Maternal Action (MAMA). Launched on Mother's Day in 2012 by then-Secretary of State Hillary Clinton, the program is a partnership between the U.S. Agency for International Development, Johnson & Johnson, the United Nations Foundation, BabyCenter, and the mHealth Alliance.

To use the free service, all a mom has to do is register by providing her due date or the birth date of her youngest child. She then receives weekly messages and reminders for the rest of her pregnancy and the first year of her baby's life. These messages include advice on nutrition, breastfeeding, newborn care, immunizations, and more. The reminders help increase the likelihood that she and her baby receive care on time. While it's too soon to tell just how much of a health impact the service has made, MAMA continues to expand. To date, it's being used in 35 countries.[172]

While MAMA is a huge, highly technical project, it doesn't always take a lot of investment or resources to make a difference. As far back as 1996, the Rural Extended Services and Care for Ultimate Emergency Relief program in Uganda taught volunteer birth attendants about the signs of pregnancy complications and then gave them the simplest of mobile tools: walkie-talkies. This enabled attendants to call for emergency transportation when they encountered a mother or baby in distress, which slashed the maternal mortality rate by half.[168]

As part of the Midwives Mobile-Phone Project in Indonesia, World Vision in 2005 provided midwives with mobile phones and phone credit so they could consult with obstetric specialists as needed. Because they could consult more frequently with more experienced physicians and staff and had access to more medical information, the midwives were better able to solve challenging health problems.[168] They could also treat more women because they could communicate via phone and only went to a patient's home when truly necessary. Collaboration improved within the healthcare system as information flowed both vertically and horizontally across the formal hierarchy. Mobile phones were also used to refer patients to the hospital when the midwives could not handle complicated medical situations.

The outcomes report on the project found that midwives felt more comfortable and confident handling deliveries because they could access expert help. "Overall," the authors wrote, "our findings confirm that (information and communication technologies) are effective in enhancing the work performance of healthcare workers and improving the efficiency of the healthcare system, proving beneficial as a capabilities enhancer...."[173]

Interventions such as the Wired Mothers project in Zanzibar suggest that mHealth has potential to improve maternal health outcomes by increasing skilled delivery attendance and access to live-saving health care interventions.[174]

A cluster randomized study of the project followed 2,550 pregnant women from their first prenatal visit to 42 days after birth. The intervention group received text messages about health education, reminders about prenatal visits and the importance of having a healthcare worker at the delivery, and information about postnatal care. The messages were customized based on the woman's gestational age throughout the pregnancy.

Sixty percent of women in the intervention group versus 47 percent in the control group delivered with skilled attendance, significantly more women had more than one prenatal visit, complication rates in the intervention group were 7.5 percent versus 11.5 percent in the control group, and maternal morbidity among the intervention group fell from nearly 500 per 100,000 live births to just under 300 between 2005 and 2009, although that is related to a variety of interventions in addition to the Wired Mothers project (Figure 6-3).[174,175]

As you can see, mHealth improves maternal and child outcomes so significantly, that the main question to ask is why it isn't being used in every country, including the United States.

Figure 6-3. Wired Mothers: Mortality Outcomes

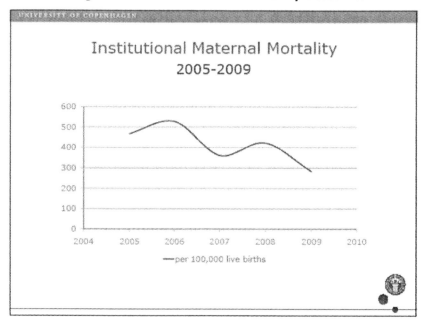

Source: Lund S, Hemed M. Wired Mothers: Use of Mobile Phones to Improve Maternal and Neonatal Health in Zanzibar. Copenhagen: University of Copenhagen. Available at: http://www.oresund.org/logistics/content/download/74534/429853/file/Ida-_Marie_Boas_Wired_Mothers.pdf. Accessed March 8, 2013.

"No matter how smart your smartphone is, it can't deliver a baby. But what it can do is provide that linkage to prevent maternal and child morbidity and mortality."

Patricia Mechael, Ph.D.,
Adjunct Assistant Professor of International and Public Affairs at Columbia
University, New York,
Speaking at the 2012 mHealth Summit.

Using mHealth to Improve Immunization Rates

The worst measles outbreak in the United States in more than 20 years occurred in 2011, with 222 confirmed cases but no deaths.[176] Compare that to the more than 100,000 children who die of measles each year around the world, most in developing countries.

While four out of five of the world's children receive the three most basic vaccines during their first year of life—diphtheria, tetanus, and pertussis—the WHO reports that 70 percent of the 22.4 million children who *don't* get those vaccines live in one of 10 countries: Afghanistan, Chad, Democratic Republic of Congo, Ethiopia, India, Indonesia, Nigeria, Pakistan, Philippines, and South Africa.[137]

That lack of protection partially explains why, in the developing world, children are 33 times more likely to die before age 5 than a child born in a developed country—all from preventable or treatable diseases and conditions like pneumonia, diarrhea, malaria, and measles.[168] If vaccine coverage worldwide increased from 2009 levels of 82 percent to just 90 percent, the WHO estimates that it would save an additional *2 million lives* a year.[177]

Enter mHealth.

mHealth reminders encourage parents to get their children vaccinated—and many of the programs listed earlier are designed to do just that. In Bangladesh, the Ministry of Health and Family Welfare made child immunizations a priority when it created a National Immunization Day more than 30 years ago. More recently, it's brought mHealth into the mix with a texting campaign to every mobile phone in the country on National Immunization Day, encouraging parents to bring their children to free immunization events and centers.[4]

In rural western Kenya, researchers enrolled 72 women in a study and sent half of them text reminders three days before and on the scheduled day of the infant's first and second immunizations. They also gave the women $2 (via cell) or provided free phone minutes to the women if their child was vaccinated within four weeks of the scheduled date. Ninety percent of the children whose mothers received the texts received the first vaccine within four weeks of the scheduled date; 86 percent received the second. That compares to just 60 percent of the children whose mothers did not receive reminders.[178]

And in Bangladesh, where almost a billion people had mobile phone subscriptions in 2012, the health ministry collects mobile phone numbers of all pregnant mothers and uses that information to send text reminders about vaccinations and to monitor the babies' vaccination rates. Immunization rates jumped 85 percent in just the first year of the program. Not surprisingly, the minister of health won the Bill and Melinda Gates Foundation's Vaccination Innovation Award for 2011.[179]

Case Study: Mapping Malaria

Positive Innovation for the Next Generation (PING) is a youth-led organization based in Botswana that implements health- and youth-related technology projects. Its goal is to address health and development problems by simultaneously using technology in an innovative way and creating more problem solvers in the local population. PING collaborated with partners at the Clinton Health Access Initiative and the Botswana Ministry of Health in a 15-month pilot from March 2011 to June 2012 to use smartphones for a Malaria Early Epidemic Detection System (MEEDS).[180]

The program enabled health facilities to submit regular reports to the Ministry of Health, give health workers the ability to report real-time disease outbreak data and tag the data with GPS

Case Study: Mapping Malaria

coordinates, and send out SMS disease outbreak alerts to all other healthcare workers in the district. Instead of the three to five weeks required with paper records, the data is reported, collected, and aggregated in minutes. Among the results:

- District and national officials were notified of all positive cases of malaria within 48 hours of diagnosis.

- An average of 77 percent of participating health facilities sent key indicator reports weekly.

- Automatically generated analysis of case report data was immediately available online to local and district health workers.

- Workers successfully mapped positive malaria cases by residence, then investigated them and monitored the patients.

- Testing for suspected malaria cases increased from 11 percent to 98.4 percent.

Way Cool: A Mobile Microscope

Aydogan Ozcan, an associate professor at UCLA, has created portable and lightweight microscopes that attach to cellphones, enabling the phones to become mobile medical labs capable of analyzing blood, bodily fluids, and water samples to diagnose potentially life-threatening diseases. The lensless microscopes are based on algorithms and computer codes that examine how light plays off the cells under investigation, then compares those patterns to ones stored in a digital database of TB, malaria, certain sexually transmitted infections, HIV, and other diseases. The cost? Ten to 15 cents per test.[181]

Teaching Doctors Through mHealth

Kenya lies 1,000 miles northeast of Malawi. Although it has the most advanced economy in the region, it is still a developing country with half its population living in poverty.

Kenya's Kijabe Hospital, two hours outside of Nairobi, is a rare gem in the region. A modern, well-equipped, and clean hospital, it employs a staff of 100 that treats 10,000 patients a month.

Until recently, however, the hospital was severely lacking in medical reference materials and healthcare technology tools. Like other hospitals in the region, much of its equipment, resources, and medicines were donated, often from hospitals in the United States that no longer needed them. While most of the equipment could be used, the old medical books were obsolete, often 60 to 80 years old.[133] There were also too few books; as many as 30 students shared six reference books.

Enter an mHealth project called Health eVillages, founded in 2011 in partnership with the Robert F. Kenney Center for Justice and Human Rights and Physicians Interactive.[182] The project provides handheld devices—iPod Touches and iPads—to healthcare professionals in the developing world. The devices arrive loaded with up-to-date medical reference materials as well as training videos and decision-making tools. Now instead of sharing a few tattered and outdated books, the medical students have access to current, evidence-based content from high-profile physicians and researchers.

It immediately made a difference. The day before the tablets arrived via Health eVillages, a patient died from complications from cancer. Yet on the day they started using the tablets, the staff treated another cancer patient with similar complications using the eVillages devices to search for treatment protocols and were able to save him.

A nurse practitioner used the tablet to study infant resuscitation in preparation for a 15-year-old girl's delivery and was able to save the baby later that day when it was born not breathing.

In Haiti, Health eVillages armed nursing educators from Massachusetts with tablets and iPod Touches loaded with clinical decision support tools and healthcare references to help train Haitian clinicians.[126]

The African Medical and Research Foundation is also using mHealth to educate health workers in Kenya and Uganda. The program allows midwives and other health workers to access a comprehensive eLearning system via their cellphones. In addition to watching virtual lectures and other educational videos, they can use the system to seek advice from colleagues and experts. Although outcome data are not available, the program was considered successful enough to be replicated in Tanzania and Zanzibar.[183]

Way Cool: Cheap Tablets, Mini "Computers"

You're not going to find $500 iPads or even $200 Kindle Fires in the hands of many people in developing nations. But you might find a $47 tablet that India's Education Ministry is producing and calling the "world's cheapest computer," or a $25 computer-on-a-stick that Britain's Raspberry Pi Foundation plans to give to children in developing countries.

Datawind, the United Kingdom-based company that developed the Indian tablet, sold its entire inventory of 30,000 Aakashes in three days and had a backlog of 1.2 million orders within two weeks. This, despite the fact that the tablet doesn't have a touch screen, runs four-year-old Android software, and has a battery life of just three hours. But wait ... analysts predict the cost may drop as low as $10 as new versions are rolled out.[123]

Long-Distance Diagnosis and Treatment

In countries where patients and specialists are separated by vast distances, mHealth is transforming the patient-doctor dynamic through the virtual world and e-diagnoses, aka, telehealth.

For instance, in China, where heart disease kills 3 million people a year, healthcare workers can simply hold a phone over sensors on a patient's chest for 30 seconds. Software in the phone collects that data and transmits it to a Beijing call center where 40 physicians work around the clock to interpret the echocardiograms and send back diagnoses.[138]

In India, where millions of people who live in rural areas have little to no access to medical centers, Apollo Hospitals Group is giving a range of devices—blood glucose testing kits, heart rate monitors, blood pressure monitors—to patients so they can measure these health indicators at home. One of the hospital's initiatives, called Sugar 24X7, allows people with diabetes to text their blood sugar readings to a health professional who then texts back information about what the readings mean and what the patient should do.[97,162]

In Zambia, which has the world's second highest cervical cancer rates and few personnel or resources to screen women with Pap tests, nurses and healthcare workers have learned to apply acetic acid (vinegar) to a woman's cervix, which causes abnormal tissue to temporarily appear white. If white tissue appears, the nurse inserts a special camera, called a digital medical scope, into the woman's vagina and snaps a photo. The images are then uploaded to a mobile phone application, and a doctor hundreds of miles away reviews them for evidence of cervical cancer. This technique has enabled 58,000 women to be screened over five years.[134,104]

While the quality of e-diagnosis isn't quite as good as the quality of real-time diagnosis, it's startlingly close. One study found that remote doctors reach the same diagnosis as on-site doctors about 77 percent of the time.[117]

Why not 100 percent? Remote physicians rely on someone else to question the patient, resulting in only partial information. Mobile-based protocols that more effectively guide healthcare workers through an intake could improve the history gathering and the accuracy of the diagnosis.

Way Cool: A Flying Eye Hospital

In the works: a completely retrofitted MD-10 aircraft stuffed with telecommunications and medical devices to provide ophthalmologic services to any country with a landing field. The Flying Eye Hospital is being developed for ORBIS International, which works in developing countries to address eye-related diseases and conditions. Although it will have its own on-board clinicians, they will use mHealth for real-time consultations, lectures, and discussions with international specialists around the world.[120]

Addressing the Pandemic: mHealth and HIV

Of all the people living with HIV/AIDs in the world, 69 percent live in sub-Saharan Africa, including 90 percent of the world's HIV-infected pregnant women and children.[185]

Yet, just 40 percent of those who need treatment get it. In most cases, that's not because the treatment isn't available but because they either aren't tested or aren't educated about the disease and the need for treatment.[186]

Enter cellphones.

In 2007, when Peter Benjamin joined Cell-Life—a not-for-profit company in Cape Town, South Africa, that develops open-source computer systems—his first task was to figure out why so many of the company's community technology projects were failing. He quickly learned that computers were not the answer. Few health centers had them. The ones that did have them couldn't keep them running in dusty remote areas with little access to electricity. Plus, even if he could overcome those problems, many people in the community wouldn't know how to use a computer if he was able to supply them with one. But he began to notice that, although they didn't own computers, at least half the people in these rural communities did own something else: a cellphone, and these phones worked more easily and had better connectivity than the typical computer.[187]

His interest in starting a cellphone-based mHealth initiative was born. But when he went to the national AIDS conference that year and spent two days walking around the exhibition hall, he couldn't find a single exhibitor promoting the use of mobile technology.[187]

No longer. Today, Cell-Life uses its proprietary data-collection platform to track, monitor, and report on a variety of HIV-related activities, from condom distribution to treatment literacy and training sessions.[135] In June 2012, it began implementing a mobile monitoring and reporting system it designed for the country's HIV Counseling and Testing Campaign and national antiretroviral treatment (ART) expansion program. It plans to counsel and test 15 million people in over 7,000 public and private facilities and help expand access to ART.

And in Nigeria, Cell-Life is piloting a free, open-source bar code–based software system to improve how pharmacists and clinicians monitor and manage ART drug dispensing and supplies. It is already being used with more than 300,000 patients.

In August 2008, an interdisciplinary team of organizations created Text to Change (TTC). It involved an SMS-based quiz that tested users' HIV/AIDS knowledge and encouraged testing and counseling. The app also alerted users to testing locations and reminded them that testing was free. When the local AIDS information center in Mbarara, Uganda, first sent the quiz to 15,000 mobile subscribers, the number of people getting tested jumped 40 percent in six weeks.[162]

A study called SMS to Test found that people who received motivational text messages were more likely to undergo an HIV test than those who didn't receive them.[136]

Project Masiluleke is a text messaging HIV/AIDS "hotline" in South Africa. Once implemented, hotline contacts jumped 350 percent since texts cost less than a penny and allowed users to ask personal questions without anyone hearing. The texting also allowed hotline attendants to answer several questions at once rather than remain on a landline with one person for many minutes. The project now sends 1 million texts a day, most of them encouraging people to get tested or treated for HIV/AIDS.[162]

Another example: When a maternity hospital in Johannesburg, South Africa, texted 386 HIV-positive mothers reminding them to give their babies ART and to show up for appointments, the percentage of mothers who took their babies for HIV testing at six weeks of age jumped from 58 percent to 74 percent.[136]

These programs are important for many reasons, but two in particular: those who test positive for HIV can begin immediate treatment as recommended, turning what used to be a death sentence into a chronic, treatable disease, and immediate treatment can reduce the risk of transmission by 96 percent.[188]

That risk reduction only occurs, however, if patients adhere to their antiretroviral treatments. Otherwise, viral loads rise and they run the risk of developing ART-resistant disease.

While studies find that ART adherence is, surprisingly, higher in developing countries than industrialized countries like the United States (one review found 77 percent adherence levels in sub-Saharan Africa compared to 55 percent in North America), it's still not where it needs to be—100 percent.[189]

To get there, AIDS organizations are turning to mHealth. In one of the first studies to evaluate the use of text-based messages for ART adherence, researchers randomized 438 adults who had just started ART to either a control group or one of four text-based intervention groups in which they received either short or long reminders sent daily or weekly.

Half the patients receiving weekly reminders achieved a 90 percent adherence rate during the 48-month follow-up compared to 40 percent of those in the control group ($P=0.03$). They were also significantly less likely to have any treatment interruptions exceeding 48 hours ($P=0.03$).[190]

As the authors wrote,

"A single server can provide text messages to thousands of patients over a wide geographic area and few human resources are needed beyond the initial setup. This strategy could be a key component of comprehensive ART adherence support."

Take Your Medicine: mHealth and Adherence

Using mHealth to improve medication adherence goes beyond texting. High-tech pill dispensers like Wisepill, contain a subscriber identity module (SIM) card that transmits a message over local cellphone networks every time the container is opened. If the dispenser remains untouched for too long, the device sends the patient a text reminder.[191] It can also send a message to healthcare workers, who can then visit the patient and try to improve adherence.

In one study of the device in South Africa, 90 percent of patients using Wisepill dispensers took their HIV medicine as directed, compared to 22 percent to 60 percent in a control group.[192]

A pilot study using a similar medication management system called SIMpill found adherence rates of 90 percent among the 130 TB patients who participated. As early as six months after the pilot, the company reported that cure rates appeared as high as 99 percent. Such an approach could be transformative in a region where directly observed treatment is the norm for both TB and HIV/AIDS, but that requires patients to visit a clinic daily to take their medication under the eye of a healthcare worker or for a healthcare worker to visit patients in their homes.

Using SIMpill, one healthcare worker can manage up to 100 patients who are self medicating. Instead of contacting all 100 patients, she just contacts the five or six who haven't taken their medications.

Way Cool: Tracking Fake Medicine

More than two-thirds of malaria medicine in Nigeria is fake or substandard. Today, however, more manufacturers are putting a strip on the packaging like the strip on a lottery card. The consumer scratches it off to reveal a unique code, uses his mobile phone to send the code to a toll-free number, and within minutes receives a text that says either "yes," meaning the drug is genuine, or "no," meaning it's a fake. The "no" message also provides a local number so the consumer can let authorities know about the fake or substandard medicine.[193]

Identifying and Overcoming Barriers

Despite the promise of mHealth in the developing world, there are numerous challenges to its widespread implementation, many of which are surprisingly similar to those in the United States.

The biggest ones are infrastructure and financing.

Although cellphone ownership has skyrocketed in the developing world, the infrastructure to support those devices is extremely fragmented, just as it is in the United States. In Uganda, for instance, when the Wisepill devices were given to 157 patients, one technical issue after another popped up. The patients all lived roughly an hour from the nearest clinic and most did not have electricity. The researchers soon learned that the ability of a wireless signal to reliably get from point A (a sensor in a pill dispenser) to point B (a server at a company in South Africa where adherence data was kept and monitored) varied widely based on the weather, power outages, cell tower issues, geographic location, and system compatibility.

The researchers then upgraded the devices to include both GPRS (general packet radio service) *and* SMS (short messaging service) technology—essentially allowing the devices to send more signals at a faster speed. If one signal failed, a backup signal could be sent. The incidence of interrupted signals dropped 80 percent.[194]

The other major barrier is financial. A 2013 report from the mHealth Alliance bemoaned the lack of "viable sustainable financial models" for mHealth. "While there are a variety of financial models currently in use for the hundreds of mHealth projects active in low and middle-income countries," the report's authors wrote, "there is general consensus that most of these projects rely too heavily on short-term grant funding from government, foundation and private-sector entities."[170]

This fragmentation also impacts the scalability and sustainability of such projects, the report finds, given the "misalignment between ecosystem players."

Who Will Pay?

The report concluded that "sustainable financial models are contingent on a deep understanding of ecosystem players, market dynamics, and each value chain members' incentives specific to each application area." Figure 6-5 depicts these value propositions. [170] Specifically:

- Applications that address medication adherence, quality monitoring, and supply chain issues and can facilitate the supply, delivery, and appropriate use of health care will appeal to private-sector players like pharmaceutical companies.

These include applications and technology to improve communication between healthcare providers, identify counterfeit drugs, and prevent clinics from running out of medications. Their appeal to the pharmaceutical industry comes from their ability to "increase and diversify revenue streams by improving their distribution logistics and the reputation of their products" as well as have a tangible impact on health outcomes.

- Applications that improve the ability of populations to access health services by addressing demand, awareness, and financial barriers should appeal to public and philanthropic-sector organizations looking to "leverage successful platforms, business models, and services from other sectors to deliver health services and information."

- Applications that address performance and accountability in health workers should induce government funding, assuming they can show value.

Using mHealth projects in Nigeria as an example, the report identified several options to achieve financial stability, including:

- Improving the perceived benefits to those financially involved in the program by attracting new buyers through additional services, revenue sharing, and monetizing other assets (such as data).

- Providing better evidence of a solution's value through monitoring and evaluation.

- Promoting reduction in perceived costs of mHealth products and services by unlocking new sources of revenue or introducing new payment models.

Figure 6-4. Common mHealth Value Propositions

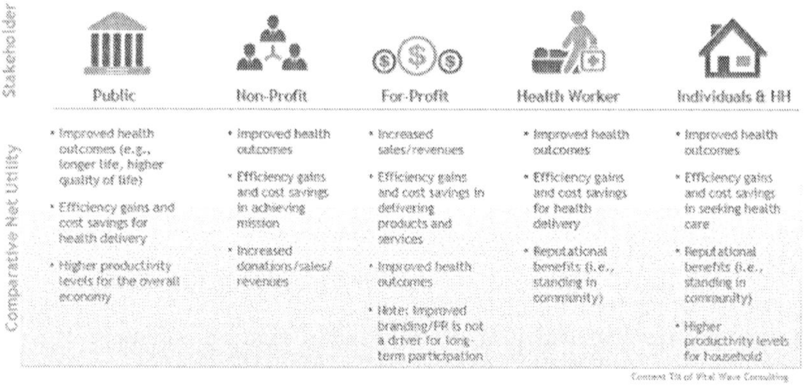

Source: "Sustainable Financing for Mobile Health (mHealth): Options and Opportunities for mHealth Financial Models in Low and Middle-Income Countries." Vital Wave Consulting and the mHealth Alliance. 2013.

Another hurdle? Just because someone owns a cellphone doesn't mean they know how to use it. Thus, researchers now know, the devices and applications for healthcare delivery in the developing world, in which much of the population is illiterate, must be simple and intuitive to use.[194]

Then there's the issue of keeping the phones charged in countries where electricity is either unavailable or unreliable. To overcome that obstacle, the developers of Text to Change distributed solar chargers with the phones. Solar-powered chargers not only power individual cellphones, but form the foundation of small businesses that buy the chargers, then sell charging time to villagers on an hourly basis.[195]

Way Cool: Charging With Dirt

Someday, cellphone owners might be able to get power from microbes in the dirt. That's the goal of a team from Harvard University that is working on a microbial fuel cell–based charger that harvests free electrons created by naturally occurring soil microbes.[196]

Another problem is cultural. In many countries, the man in the family owns and controls the phone. That can be a barrier when trying to transmit messages about pre- and postnatal care, childhood immunizations, and contraception.[136] In some Middle Eastern countries, women aren't allowed to conduct business with men, so many couldn't buy their own mobile phones. To get around that in Qatar, Vodafone gave women a red suitcase full of phones so they could host Tupperware-like parties in their homes and sell the phones to other women.[197]

Then there's scalability. Most mHealth projects to date have been small pilot projects, with just a handful expanding to the population level. Many have not been evaluated. The WHO's global survey on eHealth found that although evaluation of current mHealth pilots and programs is needed, it's not consistently being done. Just 12 percent of countries surveyed had evaluated the mHealth services already in place.[4]

To improve this dismal figure, the WHO developed its National eHealth Strategy Toolkit, a free publication available at http://www.who.int/ehealth/publications/overview.pdf. It is designed to help policy makers improve the development of a country's mHealth strategy. The comprehensive, step-by-step kit gives governments advice and tools to develop a national eHealth strategy. The kit starts by guiding governments through a visioning and goal-setting process. Then it provides a roadmap with medium- and long-term goals. It also offers ways to monitor the implementation of programs and helps governments find support and investment funds.[198]

Without such outcomes, mHealth programs are unlikely to get funding in resource-poor countries with competing priorities. Do you put limited funds into building a medical school to train doctors or buying iPads for virtual medical schools? Should you build more clinics or invest in telemedicine equipment and training? Train more health workers or improve the technology they use so they can visit more patients? These are the types of questions we expect to see answered in the coming years.

Those involved in global mHealth also need to think beyond the current focus on maternal health. More is needed in other areas, including preventing mother-to-child transmission of HIV, increasing contraception promotion and postnatal follow-up, encouraging more women to breastfeed, improving nutritional status in children, preventing and treating malaria, using insecticide-treated netting, and providing antibiotics and pediatric diarrheal treatments.[199]

Finally, despite the proliferation of mobile phones in these countries, not everyone has one. The gaps in ownership are among the people who most need access: the poorest of the poor and those with the highest rates of neonatal mortality and morbidity and infectious diseases.

Getting the Most From mHealth

Although the mHealth movement in developing countries is still young, it's old enough to have imparted some important lessons as to how we should use this technology moving forward. The following advice comes from a joint University of Washington and University of California at Berkeley review of several global mHealth projects, as well as Dr. Labrique's extensive experience.

- Use mHealth to address persistent or sharply felt problems.

- Use mHealth to strengthen a community health system that works rather than salvage one that's broken.[117]

- Develop credible programs based on sound evidence.

- Ensure programs are easy to learn and not time-consuming to use. An automated system only works if the humans who use it can handle it.

- Expect to modify any data input system over time. There's often a gap between how a system is designed and how it ends up being used. Evaluate programs so the results can be used in real-world practice and make sure they can be tested on a small-scale basis first. Identify the advantages of mHealth over current practices so potential users are convinced the costs of implementation are warranted by the benefits.

- Develop programs that are compatible with potential users' established values, norms, and facilities.

Chapter 6: Key Takeaways

✓ The developing world is more mobile than the developed world.

✓ mHealth is the *only* way the vast majority of people in the developing world will receive the health care they need given current infrastructure and resource challenges, particularly the lack of trained healthcare professionals.

✓ The promise of mHealth in the developing world lies in the sheer number of people who own cellphones.

✓ mHealth technology enables faster and easier data collection; more comprehensive training of physicians, nurses and health workers; long-distance diagnoses; educational campaigns that encourage the prevention and treatment of disease; and better communication so the people who most need medical help get it.

✓ The most important thing about mHealth is not the technology itself, but how that technology is used to improve overall health.

✓ In the developing world, even the simplest of the simple—a text message—has the potential to affect the health of millions of people.

✓ Developers of mHealth solutions for the developing world need to keep in mind the barriers, such as lack of electricity, low literacy, and limited resources for government funding.

✓ Projects need to be designed for scalability: credible, observable, relevant, relative, easy to install and understand, compatible with values and norms, and testable.

Chapter 7. Putting It All Together: Developing Your Organization's mHealth Strategy

"Healthcare organizations are forging ahead with mobile health initiatives, but they don't necessarily have a clear game plan for the programs."

Shaw G.
Many mHealth Programs Lack Focus, Direction. *FierceMobile Healthcare.*
Available at: http://www.fiercemobilehealthcare.com.

Would you add a specialized neurology unit to your hospital or develop an insurance product without conducting a careful market analysis, writing a business plan, and ensuring that the new venture meshed with your company's overall mission and strategy?

Probably not.

But nearly a quarter of healthcare organizations are pursuing mHealth with no clear strategy or driver in mind.[200] That's what Cambridge, Mass., software consulting company Medullan found when it surveyed 106 healthcare organizations, including providers, plans, pharmaceutical and device companies, and government entities, about the drivers for and barriers to its own mHealth initiatives. Nearly a fifth of all respondents and a fourth of large organizations said they had no drivers for mHealth.

Still, if we look at the survey results with a glass-half-full perspective, we see that the majority of organizations *did* have a driver, as shown in Figure 7-1.

The primary drivers for small companies (those with fewer than 1,000 employees) were cost savings and improved health outcomes. For midsized companies (those with 1,000-4,999 employees), the top driver was member/customer/patient engagement. And for companies with more than 5,000 employees, the top pick was "no driver."

Not surprisingly, a third of respondents said their key challenge in implementing mHealth was "no clear strategy," while another third named "lack of leadership." The rest cited either lack of funding or in-house skill set.

As Madullan CEO Ahmed Albaiti said in a press release about the report: "We were surprised that so many organizations would undertake mHealth initiatives without a clear driver."

"Success in mHealth requires seeing mobile applications in the context of strategic goals, operational processes, and technical architectures—the visible apps are the proverbial 'tip of the iceberg.'"

Medullan research brief
mHealth Drivers & Barriers—2012 Survey: Healthcare Overview

We are, too. As Albaiti said: "No driver and no objectives is a recipe for disaster." Again, we completely agree. Ergo, this may be the most important chapter in the book.

Caveat alert: This is not a step-by-step recipe that will result in a perfect marriage of mHealth and your organization. Just as a surgeon cannot treat two patients with the same problem the same, we do not intend to present a one-size-fits-all, homogenized version of an mHealth strategy.

However, we *can* provide a road map that will point you in the right direction and provide the tools you need to develop the right strategy.

Figure 7-1. Primary Business Driver for mHealth Initiative

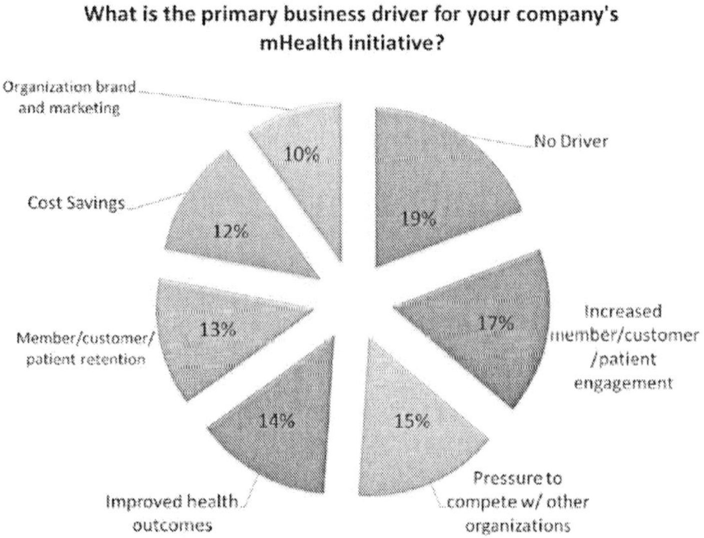

What is the primary business driver for your company's mHealth initiative?

Source: Medullan research brief. mHealth Drivers & Barriers—2012 Survey: Healthcare Overview.

Why a Strategy?

One of the best explanations for the need for a strategy and the identification of mHealth drivers in your organization comes from a report Forrester Research published in late 2012. It highlighted the results of interviews with 25 eBusiness professionals regarding best practices in scaling mobile competency.[201] Although the interviewees were not in the healthcare field, we think the challenges they identified are just as relevant for healthcare organizations:

- A lack of governance to prioritize resources

- Too little funding

- Incorrect salary bands and locations for mobile experts

- Project-based rather than enterprise-based approaches to mobile

- Inability to move as quickly as the marketplace demands

In talking with these representatives, Forrester identified the components of a strategic organization plan for mHealth:

- Cross-functional steering committee

- Center of excellence; this involves providing thought leadership and developing and distributing best practices

- Dedicated mobile development team

One theme emerged over and over: the need for collaboration between business units, vertically and horizontally throughout the organization, as well as "cross-functional collaboration to prioritize IT and mobile development resources among competing business groups."

Keep this advice in mind as you move through your own process.

Finding the Sweet Spot

"The strategy is finding the sweet spot between the business and technology drivers—and plugging in mHealth innovations into the sweet spot."'

David Shiple,
Advisory Services Practice Leader, Divurgent

The first step in developing an mHealth strategy is to review the mHealth SWOT (strengths, weaknesses, opportunities, threats) analysis and update it to reflect mHealth in your own environment.

Figure 7-2. mHealth SWOT Analysis

Strengths	Weaknesses
• Aligns with patient engagement needs • Money flowing in from investors • Technical talent coming in from other industries • Growing acceptance of online living • Smartphones becoming ubiquitous • Not contending with large legacy base • A game-changer toward the 3 aims of healthcare reform: improved experience of care, improved population health, reduced costs	• Interoperability/infrastructure • Quality of data • Many patients not engaged • Reluctance of health system to embrace wholesale change • Reimbursement for e-visits • Physicians slow to recommend mHealth products to patients
Opportunities	**Threats**
• Risk-sharing payment models, which should give home devices a positive return on investment • The "high engagement patients," especially for social media • Fast innovation cycles • Alignment with aging population preferences • Almost limitless possibilities • Likely dramatic increase in mHealth use in developing countries	• May take a while for market to shake out and stabilize • Unclear intent of large electronic health records (EHR) vendors • Failure of mHealth to "move the needle" on population health as predicted • Regulation • Political environment

Source: David Shiple, Advisory Services practice leader, Divurgent

Next, find the sweet spot. This begins with defining your business strategy, says David Shiple, who heads the Advisory Services division for the management consulting firm Divurgent. For instance, a practice manager for a large cardiology practice that is venturing into value-based purchasing as part of an accountable care organization (ACO) may have a business goal of reducing unneeded visits to its specialists.

A vendor with a home monitoring tool that can provide real-time electrocardiograms to your physicians via an iPhone could fit a business strategy, says Shiple, because it makes patients "stickier" with their doctors and provides communication and improves quality by allowing doctors to receive real-time data on patients' heart function without an office visit. This frees your physicians to treat other patients, provides early warning signs of any problems, and improves the patient experience. Under a fee-for-service model, reducing in-office visits doesn't make sense; under a bundled, shared savings, or capitated system, it does.

The next key component is the technical architecture. This defines technical standards and determines which technologies integrate with the health organization's EHRs, personal health record (PHRs), and other downstream systems.

The combination of your business strategy and technology architecture provides a filtering mechanism for the multitude of innovations in the marketplace. The next step is to build a portfolio of mHealth services that are at the intersection of your business strategy and technology architecture. Chronic disease is a good place to start given that it represents such a huge proportion of healthcare spending.

Yet, be strategic about how you integrate a chronic condition mHealth strategy into your business strategy, Shiple advises. Say you're a large health plan considering health and wellness apps for your members. Simply providing them with the app is akin to throwing a rock into the lake. You might see a few ripples, but they will fade quickly. And now your rock is gone.

However, you know that healthier members mean lower costs. So what if you tied that app to outcomes and reduced premiums or provided coupons for free copayments if patients using it improved their weight, blood sugar, or blood pressure? Now *that's* a strategic move.

Be careful, though. You don't want a tsunami of data pouring into your organization via mHealth that will overwhelm your clinicians and employees. Part of the mHealth strategy must include a discussion about how to parse the data and message it to the appropriate person, EHR, decision support rules engine, etc.

For instance, if you've provided all your congestive heart failure patients with a digital scale that can wirelessly transmit their daily weight, who gets the data? At what point does a weight gain trigger an alarm? Who receives the alarm—the doctor or nurse? How do they follow up?

These kinds of questions make mHealth strategy development and implementation similar to a chess game: you must always plan five moves ahead.

"mHealth is inevitable today because it plays into the ACO strategy: anything you can do to keep the patient in their home and out of the healthcare delivery system is good; and anything the patient can have in their hands that stops them from having to physically see their doctor is good."

David Shiple,
Advisory Services Practice Leader, Divurgent

Following the Roadmap

Now for the roadmap methodology. Let's go through each of the elements.

Figure 7-3. mHealth Strategy Methodology

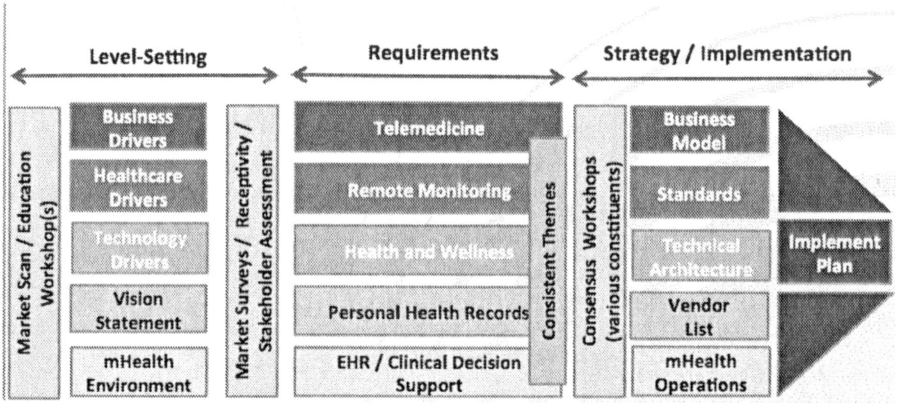

Source: David Shiple, Advisory Services practice leader, Divurgent

Level Setting

Market scan/education. Before you jump into the mHealth pool, you need to understand the true capabilities of mHealth and separate the reality from the hype. Who in your sector is doing mHealth well? Why? What does state-of-the-art mHealth look like? Where is the mHealth trajectory heading? Also important is educating your stakeholders as you move through this strategic process.

Business drivers. What are the business drivers affecting your mHealth strategy? Obvious drivers to start with include healthcare reform, ACOs, patient-centered medical homes, value-based purchasing, and meaningful use.

Healthcare drivers. This includes the relentless drive for cost savings, an aging population with more chronic conditions, and new reimbursement models that put value on fewer patient interactions—that is, keeping the patient out of the system when appropriate. Thus, there is a greater incentive to find ways to use telemedicine, home monitoring, and mHealth wellness approaches.

Technology drivers. Smaller, better, faster, cheaper technologies coupled with expanding wireless/mobile networks presents a relatively low barrier to entry for stand-alone personal health applications and devices. In addition, there is easy dissemination of apps via Apple, Google, and other distribution channels.

Vision statement. Your vision statement should encapsulate your mHealth goals and its benefits for patients and physicians. Can you develop a tagline to sum it up in a few words?

mHealth environment. How does your local market frame mHealth? For some, it is any mobile device used in health care (for example, a clinician using a smartphone to view the EHR). For others, it is home-based technologies. What should be under *your* mHealth umbrella and what shouldn't? How you define it will determine how you integrate it into your organization.

Requirements

Market survey/receptivity/stakeholder assessment. Questions to ask here include: Who are your mHealth stakeholders, what do they want, and where do they see the value? What are you willing to pay for and what do you expect patients and providers to pay for? What technologies and products are being used today by your various stakeholders, including investors, patients, and clinicians, and what is their receptivity toward future products? What about their expectations for safety, security, and privacy? Do they trust the health system?

Telemedicine. What is your organization doing in the telemedicine realm? Where could you increase its use? What are your plans for future telemedicine investment? And, also important, how receptive are your medical staff and customers to telemedicine?

Remote monitoring. Remote monitoring is one of the biggest growth areas in mHealth. But entry into this sphere requires careful consideration of your goals. What data do you want to capture? How does it get into the EHR and PHR? Who responds to the data? What modalities do your physicians and patients want? How does this monitoring intersect with your business strategy?

Health and wellness. Does it make sense to target health and wellness as an mHealth strategy? If so, where does it fit within your business model? How do you integrate it with the EHR and PHR? How do you engage the patient?

Personal health records. Do you have a PHR system and associated strategy in place and operational? How does it align with requirements for federal bonuses (i.e., meaningful use?) How does it interface with the EHR? How is patient adoption and how is it trending? Is it integrated at all with social networking and Internet search?

Electronic health record/clinical support. It is important that your mHealth efforts integrate seamlessly with the EHR. So ask if your EHR vendor has an mHealth partnership list. Find out the mHealth connectivity record with your vendor. Identify how data fed from mHealth devices can be integrated into the EHR and its clinical decision support system.

Strategy/Implementation

Consistent themes. The dimensions of mHealth will invariably overlap. For instance, remote monitoring may (and should) automatically upload to the PHR/EHR and clinical decision support programs to trigger alerts.

Consensus/workshop. Here you present the evolving mHealth model as you see it based on the work you've done in the preceding stages. Is this a viable option for your organization? Which constituents are supportive? What are alternatives? Can you reach consensus on a general business model?

Business model. Here you need to define and clarify the value proposition of mHealth for your organization; the target market and market strategy; consumer relationship; activities, resources, and personnel needed; and required core competencies. The model should also include a network/affiliation SWOT analysis, sustainability model, pro-forma analysis, high-level implementation plan, governance model, and any commercialization opportunities for proprietary systems.

Standards. What platform(s) (Windows, iOS, Android) will your system run on? This is a key filtering mechanism. If the platform doesn't integrate with your existing systems, it is a nonstarter. You must also ensure that whatever tools you adopt can "easily plug and play" into the "middleware" that will communicate data to your clinicians and to the EHR. Make sure you identify clinical standards.

Technical architecture. What are your high-level technical requirements, including hardware and software, standards, interoperability requirements, and your security and privacy needs? Are you building applications that can be run as native mobile programs (aka "apps"), or looking toward mobile Web technology that is run off a browser (Web applications, or "WAPs") ? How will you maintain version integrity as operating systems update?

Vendor list. You need to stratify your vendors and identify those most likely to help you reach your strategic goals.

mHealth operations. The roles and responsibilities of mHealth staff will be driven by your defined business model.

Implementation plan. This includes the scope of the program, funding and budget, program management, timeline, resources, risk mitigation, and a plan for change management and communications.

Spotlight on Telehealth Implementation

Telehealth is one of three legs of the mHealth stool (the other two are wellness and remote monitoring). The Commonwealth Fund synthesized findings from case studies of three early

Spotlight on Telehealth Implementation

adopters of telehealth and identified the following lessons for organizations as they implement and scale up their telehealth initiatives:[202]

- **Expect significant disruption and change in existing practices and outcomes.** An organization's ability to promote a culture of openness, preparedness, and adaptiveness to technology-led change will increase the likelihood of success.

- **Include a multidisciplinary, team-based approach.** Telehealth requires the integration of technical, clinical, and business processes into a standard program.

- **Understand that technology innovation is a social process.** Establishing leadership support and identifying program champions are the core foundations for a successful program, while patient activation and engagement are key to successful program outcomes.

- **Set low barriers to patient participation.** This includes little-to-no cost to patients and automatic enrollment.

- **Incorporate nonstandard measures into program evaluations.** These may include patient experience and staff satisfaction.

- **Scale up slowly.** It takes time to integrate technology into care delivery and to allow staff to adapt. Structure, coordination, planning, and setting goals and expectations are critical.

Lessons From the Cleveland Clinic

Here are just a few of the lessons we've learned as we develop and implement a dynamic mHealth strategy:

✓ Know your audience and what they use and want to use. For instance, in the United States, the major share of the market is held by devices on the iOS and Android operating systems. Not so in other countries, like Abu Dhabi, where we're building a new hospital and healthcare infrastructure.

✓ Understand your organizational culture and what it means for mHealth. In other words, just because you build it doesn't mean they will come (or use it). You need to first assess the willingness to change, whether that's your physicians, support staff, patients, members, or top administrators. The barriers for adoption have to be lower than the pain of adoption. On the clinical side, that means well-built, intuitive solutions that are integrated so tightly into the current workflow and technology that users barely notice them.

✓ View it from the patient perspective. We're seeing more consumer-facing apps coming into the hospital. But do developers understand the world from a hospital bed, where patients are sick, tired, scared, and in pain? We have patients who don't know how to use the call bell; will they know how to use (or want to use) tablet-based technology?

✓ Expect shorter timelines. Unlike other corporate infrastructures, which usually have a life cycle of three to five years, mobile is a different beast. It's a consumer product, and consumer-grade technologies—both software and hardware—are more fluid and dynamic with much shorter life cycles. This requires continual tinkering to keep the app up to date with platform and hardware updates.

✓ Never stop tinkering. Once you have built it, the work is not over. Content management, device upgrades, and new operating systems make mHealth a commitment. This, we find, is the "less sexy" part of mHealth: the care and feeding of what you've built.

Engaging Patients

Here are just a few of the lessons we've learned as we develop and implement a dynamic mHealth strategy:

The section above focuses on your organization. But what about the end user, who is (or should be) the patient?

The National eHealth Collaborative developed a framework for patient engagement, shown in Figure 7-4. To our minds, any mHealth strategy or app that can provide all this in an integrated manner is a winner. Think it's impossible? Just consider how well this model works for airline apps, as highlighted in Table 7-1.

Figure 7-4. National eHealth Collaborative Patient Engagement Framework

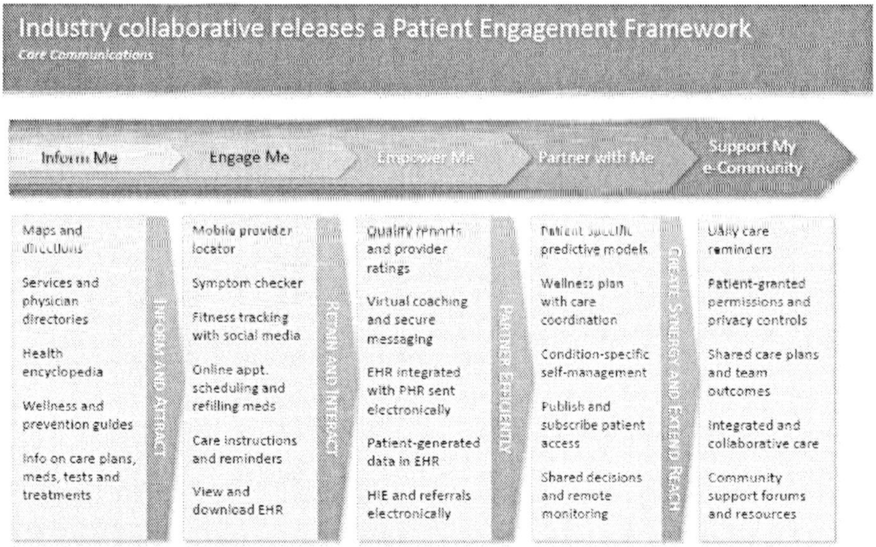

Source: National eHealth Collaborative

A report from IDC Health Insights, sponsored by AT&T, recommends that health plans and disease management organizations consider the following in developing end-to-end mHealth solutions for consumer engagement:[148]

- **Look beyond the "device and app."** Return to Figure 7-3 and ensure that your strategy includes not just the hardware and software, but intelligent back-end analytics and clinical monitoring services staffed by nurses, health coaches, and care managers.

- **Develop a scalable solution.** Supporting solutions across multiple devices, operating systems, networks, and other technological aspects requires an elaborate support system, especially in a dynamic environment where technologies are constantly evolving. You need expertise that extends beyond the existing capabilities of large healthcare organizations.

- **Ensure solutions are fully integrated.** Look beyond "cool and effective," and seek solutions that provide an integrated platform that will leverage your investment in multiple mHealth solutions and can interface with the health plan's health information databases.

- **Confirm that the solution can support multiple disease states.** mHealth strategies need to cover the entire spectrum of care, including chronic conditions as well as wellness and fitness. Long-term strategies should not require consumers to use multiple solutions to manage their various health conditions.

- **Partner wisely.** In addition to curating mHealth applications, partners can provide requisite professional services, mobile infrastructure, and support operations to provide or enable a comprehensive end-to-end solution. Partners should be carrier and technology agnostic to appeal to members using a variety of technologies (e.g., smartphone, full-featured phone, tablet, and the Internet).

Case Study: Miami Children's Hospital

Miami Children's Hospital is light years ahead of most hospitals in its implementation of mHealth, despite the fact that it only completed its strategy in 2012. Yet in 2013, the hospital won the Microsoft Health Users Group Innovation Award for Innovation in Patient Engagement for its PatientPoint Care Coordination Platform, which revolutionized the patient experience.

The hospital's transformation began with the development of its mHealth strategy in 2012. A diverse committee of stakeholders spent two months visualizing a new paradigm in patient engagement, then turning that vision into an operable process.

"The key question was 'What are we going to do from a technology standpoint to provide better care?'" and, additionally, how would their plan mesh with the changing healthcare system, explains Mallesh Murugesan, who directs Miami Children's Office of Business Development and Emerging Strategies and oversees all mHealth efforts.

To that end, they broke the patient visit into five phases: precare, before the patient enters the hospital; previsit, the time between the patient entering the hospital and receiving treatment; the care phase, when the patient is receiving care; discharge, when the patient is preparing to leave the hospital; and post-care, when the patient is back home.

"We looked at how we interface and interact with patients in each of these phases today and how we could do it tomorrow using mobile devices," Murugesan said. To visualize how this works, consider the scenario of a child who gets hurt playing soccer.

Under the old system, the mom would have to go to the emergency room, complete paperwork, and wait to be seen. Today, the mom opens the hospital's app on her phone, calls the emergency room from the app, is immediately registered, and receives a text message confirmation with a bar code. When she enters the emergency department, she scans the code into a kiosk and receives consent forms to sign, and her son is seen.

Another area addressed in the strategy planning was family interaction. To that end, Miami Children's plans to provide telemedicine or video capabilities so families can see their children wherever they are. So, continuing with the soccer example, the father, who is at work, is notified that his son is in the emergency room. He gets a link so he can videoconference with his son.

When the family leaves the hospital, the parents receive an email message with a link to a survey so they can complete it immediately, when the experience is fresh in their minds, rather than a mailed survey or phone call a couple of weeks later.

Now for post-discharge follow-up. The hospital wrote a medication adherence app called ScripteRx that both inpatient and outpatient families receive. It shows if they filled the prescription *and* sends reminders when they should take the medication. If they miss a dose, they receive a motivational message designed to encourage them to take the medication. "Medication nonadherence is a major issue here," Murugesan said, given the high population of Medicaid patients who never fill prescriptions and wind up back in the hospital.

When families return to the doctor and check in at the kiosk, they receive a message noting that they didn't fill the prescription, then are led through a series of short questions to identify the barriers to adherence. So, for instance, if the family did not fill the prescription for financial reasons, the doctor's office will provide discount coupons for their pharmacy.

"This is a perfect application," Murugesan said. "If patients take their medication, we can prevent emergency department visits, which reduces costs and improves the quality of care."

Miami Children's strategy also includes the ability to send relevant information to family phones "at the right time," such as precautions during flu season.

One reason the hospital has been able to move so quickly in these areas is that its president and CEO, M. Narendra Kini, is driving the process. "We have a CEO who thinks we should be doing a lot more than we are doing today," Murugesan said. In fact, the medication adherence app was his idea.

Part of the organization's strategy is to be completely paper-free by 2018. To that end, patients now sign consent forms and enter their personal and medical information on an iPad, which automatically uploads into the EHR.

Telemedicine: The Second Pillar

Patient engagement is one of two pillars on which Miami Children's is building its technology strategy. The other is telemedicine. To that end, the hospital developed an iPad app for secure video conferencing between physicians, which records all interactions for liability reasons. Physicians can interface with associates in the same office or link to specialists at the hospital and conduct a video consult while the patient is still in the examining room. Some offices have installed large monitors for such consultations.

The hospital is leveraging its telemedicine capabilities as a revenue generator. It developed an iPad application for area hotels. If a child gets sick, the parent enters the app, inputs information about the child, and is connected to a telemedicine coordinator who triages the call and directs the patient to a Miami Children's clinician.

The hospital also is using this method to treat children on cruise ships. As long as a medical professional is in the same room with the patient (like the nurse in the ship's sick bay), a physician in

Miami can prescribe medication. The hospital is also in discussions with several Latin American countries to provide telemedicine services.

Miami Children's isn't resting on its laurels. In 2013, it began implementing a mobile strategy to address childhood obesity in the community. "We are thinking about a gaming app that would encourage people to be healthier," Murugesan said. It is just the first of several chronic conditions the hospital plans to address through mHealth.

What Makes a Good App?

Too often we see app developers—and the institutions that embrace these apps as part of their mHealth strategy—designing apps without any thought for their usefulness. To us, the most important aspect of a good app is its integration with other apps, devices, and personal and medical health records.

There are three things an app can do: display content, perform a transaction, and communicate. A good app needs to do all three. For instance, it should display information from the patient portal; allow the patient to complete paperwork and documentation (such as entering their height, weight, and blood pressure before they arrive for an office visit); and enable the patient to communicate directly with the healthcare provider.

Airline apps have it down. With the United app, for instance, you can reserve a flight, check in for a flight, get through security, obtain a pass for the airport lounge, check your flight information (and have information about your flight pushed to you), find an airport map, see how many euros your dollars will buy, even play Sudoku and log into Facebook and Twitter—all from a single, easy-to-navigate app.

Now that's sticky.

What Makes a Good App?

Our strategy at the Cleveland Clinic is not just to regurgitate content anyone could find on a computer, but to be more strategic in what we provide. So, for example, if a patient is tracking his weight on our app and experiences a significant weight gain or loss, he would get a message to see his doctor.

Table 7-1. Customer Engagement with Airline Apps

Inform Me	Engage Me	Empower Me	Partner With Me	e-Community
Airline schedules	Check frequent flier miles	Make reservations	Upgrade me as a loyal customer	Connect to Facebook and Twitter
Airport maps	Play games	Change flights	Push flight reminders and notices of delayed or canceled flights	
Baggage costs and policies		Check in for flight	Praise employees	
Currency converter		Use as boarding pass		

Obstacles to Widespread mHealth Implementation

There are several key obstacles to widespread mHealth implementation beyond the privacy and security issues discussed in Chapter 2.

They include:

The poor quality of many apps. An investigation by the New England Center for Investigative Reporting examined 1,500 health-related apps that cost money. More than one out of five make health claims about their apps. About half the apps rely on cellphone sound, light, or vibrations for their "treatments," which, scientists interviewed by center reporters said could not possibly work for the conditions they are supposed to treat. In 2011, the Federal Trade Commission filed complaints against two developers who claimed that the light from a cellphone could cure acne. Both companies settled and paid fines.[203]

And how about a breast augmentation app from Cow Know, which claims that listening to a crying baby sound at least 20 times a day will increase a woman's breast size in the same way that breastfeeding women have larger breasts, or an app that claims it can predict the sex of a future baby?[203]

"Most of these apps are actually awful. There may be 12,000 apps out there but they're not 12,000 good apps. They're mostly bad apps that people rarely use."

Chris Wasden,
Global Healthcare Innovation Leader for PwC, speaking at MedCity Converge health tech conference, 2012

Then there are apps that purport to identify potential skin cancers from a picture. In 2013, several dermatologists wrote a letter to the editor of the *Journal of American Academy of Dermatology* expressing their concern about these apps.[204]

The doctors specifically cited the Skin Scan app, which claims to "help regular people survive their pigmentary lesions, help in diagnosis and can monitor moles over time to prevent skin cancer," and has had more than 35,000 downloads. When the app detects a high-risk nevus, it advises people to see a doctor soon. With those labeled low or medium risk, it advises them to just "keep track."

The physicians conducted their own test, using the app to analyze 93 photos of biopsy-proven melanoma. They found just a 10.8 percent sensitivity of the app to report the melanoma as high risk, with 88.2 percent of the images labeled medium risk and 1.2 percent low risk. In addition, the app often couldn't analyze the lesions despite repeated attempts.

"The potential for harm from delays in medical treatment is substantial," they wrote.

One organization seeking to improve the quality of medical apps is Happtique, a mobile health applications store and evaluation service. It released standards for testing and certifying mobile health apps in late February 2013.

The standards are designed to enable healthcare organizations to assess the content, operability, privacy, and security of mobile health apps. A panel composed of recognized leaders in mHealth, healthcare technology, healthcare certification and accreditation programs, and patient advocacy developed the standards, along with input from healthcare and information technology organizations and representatives of key federal agencies. The London-based testing and certification company Intertek will evaluate the apps and, once they pass the technical tests, send them on to medical organizations to assess their content accuracy.

Finding Financing: mHealth Start-up Incubators

Most mHealth apps and devices come from start-up companies and entrepreneurs desperate for funding. Enter the health start-up incubators Rock Health, StartUp Health, and Blueprint Health to help bridge the gap between innovation and financing.

New York-based Blueprint Health has shepherded dozens of companies through its three-month program to help them develop and launch their products. Among the nascent products in development or launched are an EHR system designed for first responders, a wristband that can tell if healthcare providers washed their hands (see "Way Cool: Did You Wash Your Hands"), and a smart pill bottle to increase adherence.

Entrepreneurs accepted into each 10-person class get $20,000 in start-up funds and three months of mentoring from healthcare professionals, insurance company executives, IT experts, and venture capitalists. Blueprint takes a 6 percent equity stake. In 2012, Blueprint had more than 1,000 applications, yet the company only accepts up to 5 percent of applicants.[205]

Mismatch between values of medical community and those of entrepreneurs. Clinicians want documented outcomes while start-ups want to get their products out there quickly and fine tune them later.[206]

Regulatory concerns. Although the U.S. Food and Drug Administration (FDA) published draft guidance in 2011 regarding regulation of medical devices and apps and, indeed, has granted 510(k) status to several, it still has not issued final rules. One of the most confusing issues is whether an app falls into the "wellness" category (and, thus, does not need approval) or the "medical" category, which requires approval. For instance, is an app that helps someone track their blood pressure and then feeds that information into the PHR a wellness app or a medical app?

"Applying a complex regulatory framework [to mobile health] could inhibit future growth and innovation in this promising market."[207]

Six members of Congress
2012 letter to the Federal Communications Commission and FDA

A year later, the House Subcommittee on Oversight and Investigations held three days of hearings on potential regulations and taxes on smartphones, tablets, mobile apps, and other healthcare technologies. During the hearing, the FDA confirmed that it had no intention of regulating smartphones or tablets, nor would it consider entities such as the iTunes app store or the Android Market or mobile platform developers to be medical device manufacturers. The agency also said it would not require that mobile medical app developers be reevaluated for minor updates, nor would it regulate apps that perform as an EHR or PHR.

That sounds nice, but it doesn't address the elephant in the room, which is the level of regulatory overview the FDA *will* impose on the apps and devices themselves. The potential for such regulation to slam the brakes on mHealth innovation is significant, in part because of the cost involved.

One estimate puts the cost of going through the approval process for a single mHealth product as high as $24 million. "Costs will go up dramatically, smaller companies will be forced out, and true innovation will slow as mHealth companies expend most of their resources on compliance," wrote Michael J. Koriwchak, M.D., of Atlanta-based ENT of Georgia, in a somewhat depressing yet possibly prescient article. "Those products that survive to reach

FDA approval will no doubt seek third-party payer reimbursement. With that will come loss of price transparency, driving up costs even further. The mHealth market will become as bloated and ineffective as the rest of the healthcare system."[163]

We can only hope he's wrong.

Way Cool: Did You Wash Your Hands

If healthcare providers simply washed their hands with hot water and soap before touching a patient or anything else, infection rates in hospitals would plummet.[205] Given that Medicare is no longer reimbursing hospitals for hospital-acquired infections, there's a huge demand for anything that can get people to the sink.

That's where IntelligentM comes in. The company has developed a bracelet that vibrates when the user has washed long enough and feeds information about the user's hand-washing habits to the employer.

Another weapon in the washing arsenal comes from BioVigil, which is developing a chemical-sensing monitor that detects soap and alcohol-based sanitizers on employee hands.[208]

Chapter 7: Key Takeaways

✓ Organizations should not embark upon mHealth without first defining a clear strategy that meshes with its mission and corporate goals.

✓ Developing that strategy requires first identifying the organization's strengths and weaknesses in the area, as well as threats and opportunities. It also requires developing strategies to overcome those weaknesses and address those threats.

✓ Any effort to develop an mHealth strategy must involve a diverse group of stakeholders.

✓ The strategy should serve as a filtering mechanism to determine which products make the most sense for your organization.

✓ An mHealth strategy begins with level setting, moves into technology and clinical requirements, and ends with final strategy and implementation.

✓ Consumer engagement should be a core element of any mHealth strategy.

Conclusion

From the time the first human uttered a sound and another human responded, communication has been at the heart of all interactions. Nowhere is that communication been more vital than in medicine. For despite the information we can obtain from sophisticated tests, surgeries, and imaging, the most important component of any diagnostic evaluation and the greatest predictor of successful treatment is the patient/provider relationship and how the two communicate.

Yet our current system requires that these interactions occur almost exclusively in person, face-to-face, in a time-consuming, expensive, often frustrating manner that leaves neither party happy. They involve paperwork (yes, on actual paper), waiting, hurried visits, missed information, and uncoordinated follow up. The process itself interferes with the relationship, impacts the quality of the care delivered and the health of the patient, and winds up costing the system billions in waste.

The initial implementation of electronic health records and related technology has had a decidedly mixed impact on this situation. In some cases, this first generation of technology has enhanced information flow, communication and collaboration. But in far too many cases, these systems have "gotten in the way" of clinical care, degrading communication and interfering with human interaction.

mHealth has the power to change all this.

As we've tried to convey in this book, mHealth has the potential to broadly transform every aspect of health care, from how we maintain our health to how we provide care to how we pay for care. This transformation has already started. Today, wireless networks, computers, tablets, and smartphones are the "bricks and mortar" of an increasingly virtual healthcare system. Combine that with more thoughtful design and greater attention to human factors engineering and workflow, and you have a next generation of high performance tools and processes that will let the technology serve providers and patients rather than the other way around.

mHealth gives us the ability to capture reams of data and sift through that data for patterns and clues whether one is in a hospital or office – or in an African village with limited electricity and few paved roads.

It enables us to examine a patient from thousands of miles away—including looking in her ears, down her throat, and listening to her heart, and to perform an ultrasound with no more than a smartphone.

It also gives us the ability, as healthcare consumers, to take control of our own health in ways that no other form of information and communication can. To monitor our own vital signs, review our own records, and track our own health no matter where we are or what we're doing.

Most important, however, is that mHealth has the power to instantly connect healthcare consumers and providers in deep, rich, meaningful ways regardless of physical location.

Challenges Ahead

We have no choice but to embrace this tsunami of change. In developed nations, we need mHealth to help repair broken healthcare systems in which cost and quality are diametrically opposed; in which the increasing complexity of chronic disease is straining existing resources and robbing patients of quality of life. In the developing world, we need mHealth to build healthcare systems where none currently exist and to deliver quality care to exploding populations in countries with few assets and little infrastructure.

The path ahead may be clear, but it will be anything but easy. As we have highlighted throughout the book, there are many twists and turns, subtleties and barriers. In the United States alone, where health care makes up nearly 20 percent of the economy, powerful, entrenched and highly motivated stakeholders are clinging to their fax machines, paper records, and face-to-face interactions, reluctant to give up what they know for what might be. Thankfully, there are just as many of us on the other side who are willing to pry their fingers from the past and partner with them to create the future.

We are at the beginning of the beginning, much like the Model T was the beginning of the automobile age. The transformation that moved our world from one dominated by horses and buggies, where a person might never travel more than 50 miles outside his home, to one in which superhighways define our landscape and we think nothing of driving 50 miles just to have lunch, required an unprecedented partnership between consumers, industry, and government. It led to the demise of other industries (anyone need a buggy whip these days?). It was painful and exciting, and transformative.

The transformation of health care through mHealth will be similar.

At the end of the day, however, this transformation is not about bits and bytes, cool apps and hardware, or Big Data. It is about using high tech to enhance high touch because health care is different from any other industry. It is not about things, but about people. It is about how we care for each other and how we connect under some of the most joyous or most difficult times in our lives.

The rollout of mHealth must occur in a courageous and thoughtful way that appropriately balances science with art, efficiency with caring, empowerment with partnership, and optimism with realistic expectations.

We are so fortunate to live in this time of great change. We have within our reach the tools to transform health care as never before and leave an awesome legacy for future generations. But we must never forget that at the heart of all of this is just that: our hearts and their desire to heal and be healed.

Index

References

1. Ackerman K. mHealth: Closing the Gap Between Promise and Adoption. *iHealth Beat.* 2011. http://www.ihealthbeat.org/features/2011/mhealth-closing-the-gap-between-promise-and-adoption.aspx. Accessed November 12, 2012.

2. Atallah L, Jonesy GG, Ali R, et al. Observing Recovery from Knee-Replacement Surgery by using Wearable Sensors. Paper presented at: 8th International Conference on Body Sensor Networks2011; Dallas, TX.

3. HIMSS. Definitions of mHealth. 2012; http://www.mhimss.org/resource/definitions-mhealth. Accessed November 12, 2012.

4. World Health Organization. *mHealth: New horizons for health through mobile technologies.* 2011.

5. McBeth PB, Crawford I, Blaivas M, et al. Simple, almost anywhere, with almost anyone: remote low-cost telementored resuscitative lung ultrasound. *J Trauma.* Dec 2011;71(6):1528-1535.

6. HIMSS Analytics. *2nd Annual HIMSS Mobile Technology Survey.* 2012.

7. Jahns RG. The market for mHealth app services will reach $26 billion by 2017. *research2guidance.* March 7, 2013. http://www.research2guidance.com/the-market-for-mhealth-app-services-will-reach-26-billion-by-2017/. Accessed July 10, 2013.

8. Taitsman JK, Grimm CM, Agrawal S. Protecting Patient Privacy and Data Security. *N Eng J Med.* February 27, 2013.

9. Ranck J. Mobile Operators and Digital Health. *Mobihealthnews 2012 report*: Chester Street Publishing; 2012.

10. iData Research. U.S. Market for Patient Monitoring Devices. 2012; http://www.idataresearch.com/u-s-market-for-patient-monitoring-devices-2012/?r=y.

11. Dolan B. Mobile health sensor market to hit $5.6B by 2017. *Mobile Health News.* April 24, 2013. http://mobihealthnews.com. Accessed April 25, 2013.

12. Miliard M. Frost & Sullivan spotlights top opportunities for telehealth growth. *Healthcare IT News.* October 28, 2012. http://www.healthcareitnews.com/news/frost-sullivan-

spotlights-top-opportunities-telehealth-growth. Accessed November 2, 2012.

13.   Morgan SA, Agee NH. Mobile Healthcare. *Front Health Serv Manage.* 2012;29(2):3-10.

14.   Mayne L, Girod C, S. W. *2012 Milliman Medical Index.* 2012.

15.   University of Oxford. mHealth could have potential cost saving of £750 million for NHS. http://www.ibme.ox.ac.uk/news-events/news/mhealth-could-have-potential-cost-saving-of-a3750-million-for-nhs. Accessed May 26, 2013.

16.   Juniper Research. Cost Savings from Mobile Health Monitoring to Reach $1.9 billion to $5.8 Billion Globally by 2014 says Juniper Research [press release]. 2010; http://www.juniperresearch.com/viewpressrelease.php?pr=172. Accessed May 24, 2013.

17.   Accenture. *Still waiting for mHealth? Mobile devices create new opportunity in healthcare.* 2012.

18.   Boston Consulting Group and Telenor Group. *Socio-Economic Impact of mHealth.* 2012.

19.   West D. *Issues in Technology Innovation: How Mobile Devices are Transforming Healthcare.* The Brookings Institution;2012.

20.   Kulshreshtha A, Kvedar JC, Goyal A, et al. Use of remote monitoring to improve outcomes in patients with heart failure: a pilot trial. *Int J Telemed Appl.* 2010;2010:870959.

21.   Dawson A, Cohen D, Candelier C, et al. Domiciliary midwifery support in high-risk pregnancy incorporating telephonic fetal heart rate monitoring: a health technology randomized assessment. *J Telemed Telecare.* 1999;5(4):220-230.

22.   Rees RS, Bashshur N. The effects of TeleWound management on use of service and financial outcomes. *Telemed J E Health.* Dec 2007;13(6):663-674.

23.   Steventon A, Bardsley M, Billings J, et al. Effect of telehealth on use of secondary care and mortality: findings from the Whole System Demonstrator cluster randomised trial. *BMJ (Clinical research ed.).* 2012;344:e3874.

24.   van Os-Medendorp H, Koffijberg H, Eland-de Kok PC, et al. E-health in caring for patients with atopic dermatitis: a randomized controlled cost-effectiveness study of internet-guided monitoring and online self-management training. *Br J Dermatol.* May 2012;166(5):1060-1068.

25.   Medtronic. Medtronic Launches CareLink Express™ Service: Pilot
       Shows New Remote Monitoring Service Allows Quick Access to
       Care for Patients [press release]. August 14, 2012;
       http://wwwp.medtronic.com/Newsroom/NewsReleaseDetails.do
       ?itemId=1344869505352&lang=en_US. Accessed November 13,
       2012.

26.   Clemens NA. Privacy, consent, and the electronic mental health
       record: The Person vs. the System. *J Psychiatr Pract.*
       2012;18(1):46-50.

27.   Johnson A. The Do-It-Yourself House Call. *Wall St J.* July 27, 2010.

28.   Globalworkplaceanalytics.com. Latest Telecommuting Statistics.
       2012;
       http://www.globalworkplaceanalytics.com/telecommuting-
       statistics. Accessed November 11, 2012.

29.   Litan RE. *Vital Signs via Broadband: Remote Health Monitoring
       Transmits Savings, Enhances Lives.* Better Health Care
       Together;2008.

30.   Price Waterhouse Cooper. *Emerging mHealth: Paths for Growth.*
       June 2012.

31.   International Telecommunications Union. ICT Data and Statistics:
       Mobile Cellphone Telephony. 2012; http://www.itu.int/ITU-
       D/ict/statistics/. Accessed November 9, 2012.

32.   Fox S, Duggan M. *Mobile Health 2012.* Pew Internet & American
       Life Project;2012.

33.   Number of people with diabetes increases to 24 million: estimates
       of diagnosed diabetes now available for all U.S. counties [press
       release]. June 24, 2008;
       http://www.cdc.gov/media/pressrel/2008/r080624.htm.
       Accessed July 3, 2013.

34.   Number of Americans with diabetes projected to double or triple
       by 2050: older, more diverse population and longer lifespans
       contribute to increase [press release]. Atlanta, GA: Centers for
       Disease Control and Prevention; October 22, 2010.
       http://www.cdc.gov/media/pressrel/2010/r101022.html.
       Accessed July 3, 2013.

35.   Levin D. EMR & Personalized Health: "Keeping it Real" in the
       Clinical Setting. Paper presented at: Cleveland Clinic 2012
       Personalized Healthcare Summit: Personalized Healthcare for the
       Practicing Clinician. May 2012.

36. International Diabetes Federation. The Global Burden. *JDF Diabetes Atlas*. 2012.

37. eHealth Initiative. *An Issue Brief on eHealth Tools and Diabetes Care for Socially Disadvantaged Populations.* California HealthCare Foundation;2012.

38. Health and Human Services. mHealth Initiatives. 2011; http://www.hhs.gov/open/initiatives/mhealth/. Accessed November 13, 2012.

39. Federal Communications Commission. *mHealth Task Force: Findings and Recommendations.* 2012.

40. Gold J. FDA regulators face daunting task as health apps multiply. *Kaiser Health News.* June 27, 2012.

41. O'Harrow R. Health-care sector vulnerable to hackers, researchers say. *Washington Post.* December 25, 2013.

42. Shaw G. 4 Health Privacy Threats That Will Freak You Out. January 7, 2013. http://www.fiercehealthit.com/story/4-data-and-privacy-threats-will-freak-you-out/2013-01-07. Accessed January 19, 2013.

43. Lucille Packard Children's Hospital at Stanford. Notice and Frequently Asked Questions About a Recent Laptop Theft 2013; http://www.lpch.org/aboutus/news/for-patients.html. Accessed March 14, 2013.

44. Office of Inspector General, Veteran's Administration. *Review of Alleged Transmission of Sensitive VA Data Over Internet Connections.* March 6, 2013.

45. Mearian L. 'Wall of Shame' exposes 21M medical record breaches. *Computerworld.* August 7, 2012. http://www.computerworld.com/s/article/9230028/ Wall_of_Sh ame_exposes_21M_medical_record_breaches. Accessed May 12, 2013.

46. Ponemon Institute. *Third Annual Benchmark Study on Patient Privacy & Data Security.* December 2012.

47. Australian Government Department of Defense. Multi-Factor Authentication. 2013; http://www.dsd.gov.au/publications/csocprotect/multi_factor_a uthentication.htm.

48. Yu R. Lost Cellphones Added Up Fast in 2011. *USA Today.* March 23, 2012.

49.   Scherer M. Law Enforcement Sounds Alarm on Cell-Phone-Theft Epidemic. *Time.* March 25, 2013.

50.   Health and Human Services. Breaches Affecting 500 or More Individuals. 2012; http://www.hhs.gov/ocr/privacy/hipaa/administrative/breachnotificationrule/breachtool.html. Accessed May 13, 2013.

51.   HitConsultant. 3 Basics of Effective BYOD for Your Healthcare Organization. February 12, 2013. http://www.hitconsultant.net/2013/02/12/3-basics-of-effective-byod-for-your-healthcare-organization/. Accessed March 14, 2013.

52.   Jackson S. 8 strategies for tightening mobile security at hospitals. *FierceMobileHealthcare.* July 22, 2011. http://www.fiercemobilehealthcare.com/story/8-strategies-tightening-mobile-security-hospitals/2011-07-22. Accessed May 13, 2013.

53.   Kirk J. Pacemaker Hack Can deliver Deadly 830-volt Jolt. *NetworkWorld.* October 17, 2012. http://www.networkworld.com/news/2012/101712-pacemaker-hack-can-deliver-deadly-263445.html. Accessed March 15, 2013.

54.   United States General Accounting Office. *Medical Devices: FDA Should Expand Its Consideration of Information Security for Certain Types of Devices.* 2012.

55.   Marcus AD, Weaber C. Heart Gadgets Test Privacy-Law Limits. *Wall St J.* November 28, 2012.

56.   McGraw D, Pfister HR, Ingargiola SR, Belfort RD. Lessons from Project HealthDesign: Strategies for Safeguarding Patient-Generated Health Information Created or Shared through Mobile Devices. *J Healthcare Inform Manag.* Summer 2012;26(3):24-29.

57.   Acohido B. Anti-virus firms push security software for mobile devices. *USA Today.* September 19, 2011.

58.   Mosquera M. mHealth Stakeholders Await Clarity Across Regulatory Landscape. *mHIMSS.* November 26, 2012. http://tinyurl.com/aejrk76. Accessed November 29, 2012.

59.   Happtique Unveils Final Standards for Certifying Mobile Health Apps. *iHealth Beat.* February 28, 2013. http://www.ihealthbeat.org/articles/2013/2/28/happtique-unveils-final-standards-for-certifying-mobile-health-apps.aspx. Accessed March 15, 2013.

60.   US Department of Health and Human Services. *Managing Mobile Devices in Your Health Care Organization.*

61.   Karasz HN, Eiden A, Bogan S. Text Messaging to Communicate With Public Health Audiences: How the HIPAA Security Rule Affects Practice. *Am J Public Health.* Apr 2013;103(4):617-622.

62.   Quinn CC, Shardell MD, Terrin ML, Barr EA, Ballew SH, Gruber-Baldini AL. Cluster-randomized trial of a mobile phone personalized behavioral intervention for blood glucose control. *Diabetes Care.* Sep 2011;34(9):1934-1942.

63.   WellDoc. The WellDoc® DiabetesManager® Cuts Hospital and ER Visits in Half [press release]. December 6, 2011; http://www.businesswire.com/news/home/20111206005830/en. Accessed December 25, 2012.

64.   Centers for Disease Control and Prevention. 2011 National Diabetes Fact Sheet. http://www.cdc.gov/diabetes/pubs/estimates11.htm. Accessed December 24, 2012.

65.   Shaw JE, Sicree RA, Zimmet PZ. Global estimates of the prevalence of diabetes for 2010 and 2030. *Diabetes Res Clin Pract.* Jan 2010;87(1):4-14.

66.   Christensen C, Bohmer R, Kenagy J. Will disruptive innovations cure healthcare? *Harv Bus Rev.* Vol 782000:102-112, 199.

67.   Christensen CM. A disruptive solution for health care. 2011; http://blogs.hbr.org/innovations-in-health-care/2011/03/a-disruptive-solution-for-heal.html. Accessed December 7, 2012.

68.   Ryan K. Texting Among Doctors Raises Privacy Concerns. *Hispanic Business.* November 13, 2012. http://www.hispanicbusiness.com/2012/11/13/texting_among_doctors_raises_privacy_concerns.htm. Accessed December 23, 2012.

69.   *Point-of-care computing for nursing.* Spyglass Consulting Group;November 2012.

70.   Farnan JM, Snyder Sulmasy L, Worster BK, et al. Online medical professionalism: patient and public relationships: policy statement from the American College of Physicians and the Federation of State Medical Boards. *Ann Intern Med.* Apr 16 2013;158(8):620-627.

71.   Kellermann AL, Jones SS. What it will take to achieve the as-yet-unfulfilled promises of health information technology. *Health Aff (Millwood).* Jan 2013;32(1):63-68.

72. Abbass I, Helton J, Mhatre S, Sansgiry SS. Impact of electronic health records on nurses' productivity. *Comput Inform Nurs.* May 2012;30(5):237-241.

73. Abelson R, Creswell J, Palmer G. Medicare bills rise as records turn electronic. *New York Times.* September 21, 2012.

74. Phansalkar S, van der Sijs H, Tucker AD, et al. Drug-drug interactions that should be non-interruptive in order to reduce alert fatigue in electronic health records. *J Am Med Inform Assoc.* May 1 2013;20(3):489-493.

75. Embi PJ, Leonard AC. Evaluating alert fatigue over time to EHR-based clinical trial alerts: findings from a randomized controlled study. *J Am Med Inform Assoc.* Jun 2012;19(e1):e145-148.

76. Wrenn JO, Stein DM, Bakken S, Stetson PD. Quantifying clinical narrative redundancy in an electronic health record. *J Am Med Inform Assoc.* Jan-Feb 2010;17(1):49-53.

77. Thornton JD, Schold JD, Venkateshaiah L, Lander B. Prevalence of copied information by attendings and residents in critical care progress notes. *Crit Care Med.* Feb 2013;41(2):382-388.

78. Freudenheim M. The Ups and Downs of Electronic Medical Records. *New York Times.* October 8, 2012.

79. Mace S. How Tablets are Influencing Healthcare. *HealthLeaders.* March 6, 2013. http://www.healthleadersmedia.com/print/TEC-289831/How-Tablets-are-Influencing-Healthcare. Accessed May 2, 2013.

80. Reed M, Huang J, Graetz I, et al. Outpatient electronic health records and the clinical care and outcomes of patients with diabetes mellitus. *Ann Intern Med.* Oct 2 2012;157(7):482-489.

81. Palen TE, Ross C, Powers JD, Xu S. Association of online patient access to clinicians and medical records with use of clinical services. *JAMA.* Nov 21 2012;308(19):2012-2019.

82. Walker JM, Hassol A, Bradshaw B, Rezaee ME. *Health IT Hazard Manager Beta-Test: Final Report.* Rockville, MD: Agency for Healthcare Research and Quality;May 2012.

83. Carayon P, Karsh B. *Incorporating Health Information Technology Into Workflow Redesign.* Rockville, MD: Agency for Healthcare Research and Quality. October 2012.

84. Committee on Patient Safety and Health Information Technology. *Health IT and Patient Safety: Building Better Systems for Better Care.* Washington, DC. 2011.

85.   Burnett M, et al. A simple, real-time text-messaging intervention is associated with improved door-to-needle times for acute ischemic stroke. Paper presented at: American Academy of Neurology2013; San Diego, CA.

86.   Bodenheimer T, Lorig K, Holman H, Grumbach K. Patient self-management of chronic disease in primary care. *JAMA.* Nov 20 2002;288(19):2469-2475.

87.   Lorig K, Ritter PL, Laurent DD, et al. Online diabetes self-management program: a randomized study. *Diabetes Care.* Jun 2010;33(6):1275-1281.

88.   Lorig K, Alvarez S. Re: Community-based diabetes education for Latinos. *Diabetes Educ.* Jan-Feb 2011;37(1):128.

89.   Robert Wood Johnson Foundation. When Patients Share Health Info with Providers Through Personal Technologies, Clinical Care and Patient Engagement Improve. September 26, 2012; http://rwjf.org/en/about-rwjf/newsroom/newsroom-content/2012/09/When-Patients-Share-Health-Info-with-Providers-through-Personal-Technologies-Clinical-Care-and-Patient-Engagement-Improve.html. Accessed December 22, 2012.

90.   Chase D. Xboxification of Healthcare. *Forbes.* December 4, 2012.

91.   McNickle M. 7 E-Health Tools to Get Patients Engaged. *Information Week.* October 8, 2012. http://www.informationweek.com/healthcare/patient/7-e-health-tools-to-get-patients-engaged/240008652?pgno=5. Accessed December 22, 2012.

92.   Khan S, Maclean CD, Littenberg B. The effect of the Vermont Diabetes Information System on inpatient and emergency room use: results from a randomized trial. *Health Outcomes Res Med.* Jul 2010;1(1):e61-e66.

93.   Littenberg B, MacLean CD, Zygarowski K, Drapola BH, Duncan JA, Frank CR. The Vermedx Diabetes Information System reduces healthcare utilization. *Am J Manag Care.* Mar 2009;15(3):166-170.

94.   Maclean CD, Gagnon M, Callas P, Littenberg B. The Vermont diabetes information system: a cluster randomized trial of a population based decision support system. *J Gen Intern Med.* Dec 2009;24(12):1303-1310.

95.   McNickle M. Patient Engagement Tools Reduce Hospital Readmission Rates. *Information Week.* September 27, 2012. http://www.informationweek.com/healthcare/patient/patient-

engagement-tools-reduce-hospital/240008088. Accessed
December 22, 2012.

96.   Rothemich SF, Massoudi B. BreathEasy: A Smartphone PHR for
       Patients with Asthma. 2012;
       http://www.allhealth.org/briefingmaterials/Rothemich-
       BreathEasy-2367.pdf. Accessed December 22, 2012.

97.   mHealth team for PwC. *Emerging mHealth: Paths for Growth.* June
       2012.

98.   Peck AD. App-solutely fabulous: Mobile health apps on the rise.
       Medical Economics. November 25, 2011.
       http://medicaleconomics.modernmedicine.com/memag/article/
       articleDetail.jsp?id=752524&sk=&date=&pageID=2. Accessed
       November 29, 2012.

99.   Jencks SF, Williams MV, Coleman EA. Rehospitalizations among
       patients in the Medicare fee-for-service program. *N Eng J Med.* Apr
       2 2009;360(14):1418-1428.

100.   Lemieux J, Sennett C, Wang R, Mulligan T, Bumbaugh J. Hospital
       readmission rates in Medicare Advantage plans. *Am J Manag Care.*
       Feb 2012;18(2):96-104.

101.   Konschak C, Flareau B. New Frontiers in Home Telemonitoring.
       It's Already Here; Where are You? *JHIM.* 2008;22(2):16-23.

102.   Chumbler NR, Neugaard B, Ryan P, Qin H, Joo Y. An observational
       study of veterans with diabetes receiving weekly or daily home
       telehealth monitoring. *J Telemed Telecare.* 2005;11(3):150-156.

103.   Jacob S. THR Pilot Study: Wireless Monitoring Cuts Heart Failure
       Readmissions by 27 Percent. *DHealthcare Daily.* 2012.
       http://healthcare.dmagazine.com/2012/08/13/thr-pilot-study-
       wireless-monitoring-cuts-heart-failure-readmissions-by-27-
       percent/. Accessed November 29, 2012.

104.   Graham J, Tomcavage J, Salek D, Sciandra J, Davis DE, Stewart WF.
       Postdischarge monitoring using interactive voice response
       system reduces 30-day readmission rates in a case-managed
       Medicare population. *Medical Care.* Jan 2012;50(1):50-57.

105.   Sorknaes AD, Madsen H, Hallas J, Jest P, Hansen-Nord M. Nurse
       tele-consultations with discharged COPD patients reduce early
       readmissions--an interventional study. *Clin Respir J.* Jan
       2011;5(1):26-34.

106.   Wicklund E. Kentucky physician touts advantages of house calls
       by smartphone. *mHIMSS.* March 15, 2013.

http://www.mhimss.org/news/kentucky-physician-touts-advantages-house-calls-smartphone. Accessed March 21, 2013.

107. Switzer JA, Demaerschalk BM, Xie J, Fan L, Villa KF, Wu EQ. Cost-Effectiveness of Hub-and-Spoke Telestroke Networks for the Management of Acute Ischemic Stroke From the Hospitals' Perspectives. *Circ Cardiovasc Qual Outcomes.* Dec 4 2013;6(1):18-26.

108. Baker LC, Johnson SJ, Macaulay D, Birnbaum H. Integrated telehealth and care management program for Medicare beneficiaries with chronic disease linked to savings. *Health Aff (Millwood).* Sep 2011;30(9):1689-1697.

109. McCann E. Remote monitoring savings pegged at $1.4M for Dartmouth Hitchcock. *Healthcare IT News.* June 18, 2012. http://www.healthcareitnews.com/news/savings-remote-monitoring-pegged-14m-dartmouth-hitchcock

110. Dansky KH, Palmer L, Shea D, Bowles KH. Cost analysis of telehomecare. *Telemed J E Health.* Fall 2001;7(3):225-232.

111. Bertakis KD, Azari R. Patient-centered care is associated with decreased health care utilization. *J Am Board of Fam Med.* May-Jun 2011;24(3):229-239.

112. Pew Internet and American Life Project. Pew Internet: Mobile. 2012; http://pewinternet.org/Commentary/2012/February/Pew-Internet-Mobile.aspx. Accessed April 24, 2013.

113. Caine K, Hanania R. Patients want granular privacy control over health information in electronic medical records. *J Am Med Inform Assoc.* Jan 1 2013;20(1):7-15.

114. Wolters Kluwer Health. *Wolters Kluwer Health Quarterly Poll: Consumerization of Healthcare.* 2012.

115. Anania Communications Regulatory Authority. Quarterly Statistics: Dar es Salaam. 2013; http://www.tcra.go.tz/index.php/quarterly-telecommunications-statistics#. Accessed March 1, 2013.

116. Kearney AT. Improving the Evidence for Mobile Health. 2012; http://www.gsma.com/connectedliving/wp-content/uploads/2012/03/atkearneyevidenceformobilehealthwhitepaper.pdf. Accessed February 26, 2013.

117. Derenzi B, Borriello G, Jackson J, et al. Mobile phone tools for field-based health care workers in low-income countries. *Mt Sinai J Med.* May-Jun 2011;78(3):406-418.

118. World Health Organization. Global Health Observatory. Infant mortality: situation and trends. 2013; http://www.who.int/gho/child_health/mortality/neonatal_infant_text/en/index.html. Accessed March 2, 2013.

119. Centers for Disease Control and Prevention. Fast Stats: Therapeutic Drug Use. 2011; http://www.cdc.gov/nchs/fastats/drugs.htm. Accessed April 24, 2013.

120. Wicklund E. mHealth technology used to develop "Flying Eye Hospital". *mHIMSS.* 2013. http://www.mhimss.org/news/mhealth-technology-used-develop-flying-eye-hospital. Accessed March 21, 2013.

121. mobiThinking. Global mobile statistics 2013 Part A: Mobile subscribers; handset market share; mobile operators. 2012; http://mobithinking.com/mobile-marketing-tools/latest-mobile-stats/a. Accessed May 8, 2013.

122. Horvath T, Azman H, Kennedy GE, Rutherford GW. Mobile phone text messaging for promoting adherence to antiretroviral therapy in patients with HIV infection. *The Cochrane database of systematic reviews.* 2012;3:CD009756).

123. Smith M. India's sub-$50 Android tablet claims 1.4 million orders in two weeks. *engadget.* January 4, 2012. http://www.engadget.com/2012/01/04/india-sub-50-android-tablet-1-4-million-orders/. Accessed March 18, 2013.

124. Al-Adhroey AH, Nor ZM, Al-Mekhlafi HM, Mahmud R. Opportunities and obstacles to the elimination of malaria from Peninsular Malaysia: knowledge, attitudes and practices on malaria among aboriginal and rural communities. *Malar J.* 2010;9:137.

125. PwC. Value: Getting it. Giving it. Growing it. *Communications Review.* 2010;15(3):1-48.

126. Wicklund E. Health eVillages launches new mHealth effort in Haiti. 2013. http://www.mhimss.org/news/health-evillages-launches-new-mhealth-effort-haiti. Accessed March 17, 2013.

127. Burke LE, Styn MA, Sereika SM, et al. Using mHealth technology to enhance self-monitoring for weight loss: a randomized trial. *Am J Prev Med.* Jul 2012;43(1):20-26.

128. Wicklund E. A 'disaster doc' offers his take on mHealth's advantages. *mHIMSS.* April 15, 2013.

http://www.mhimss.org/news/disaster-doc. Accessed April 16, 2013.

129. Mathews AW. Doctors Move to Webcams. *Wall St J.* December 20, 2012.

130. Arora S, Peters AL, Agy C, Menchine M. A mobile health intervention for inner city patients with poorly controlled diabetes: proof-of-concept of the TExT-MED program. *Diabetes Technology & Therapeutics.* Jun 2012;14(6):492-496.

131. Brownlee C. mHealth – Can You Hear Me Now? *The Magazine of the Johns Hopkins University Bloomberg School of Public Health.* 2012. http://magazine.jhsph.edu/2012/technology/features/mHealth/page_1/. Accessed January 13, 2013.

132. Shapiro JR, Bauer S, Andrews E, et al. Mobile therapy: Use of text-messaging in the treatment of bulimia nervosa. *Int J Eat Disord.* Sep 2010;43(6):513-519.

133. Linder M. African Teaching Hospital Gets Ahead with Skyscape Apps. http://www.healthevillages.org/news-from-the-field/african-teaching-hospital-gets-ahead-with-skyscape-apps/. Accessed February 25, 2013.

134. Mwanahamuntu MH, Sahasrabuddhe VV, Kapambwe S, et al. Advancing cervical cancer prevention initiatives in resource-constrained settings: insights from the Cervical Cancer Prevention Program in Zambia. *PLoS Med.* May 2011;8(5):e1001032.

135. Phippart T. The (M)Health Connection: An Examination Of The Promise Of Mobile Phones For HIV/AIDS Intervention In Sub-Saharan Africa [master's thesis]. 2012; ir.lib.uwo.ca/cgi/viewcontent.cgi?article=1962&context=etd. Accessed February 27, 2013.

136. Donner J, Mechael P. *MHealth in Practice: Mobile Technology for Health Promotion in the Developing World.* New York: Bloomsbury Academic; 2013.

137. World Health Organization. Immunization Highlights. 2012; http://www.who.int/immunization/newsroom/highlights/2012/en/index1.html. Accessed March 2, 2013.

138. Qualcomm Wireless Reach Initiative. The Computerworld Honors Program: honoring those who use information technology to benefit society. December 2011; www.cwhonors.org/case_studies/2012Finalists/Health/2919.pdf. Accessed March 3, 2013.

139. World Bank. 2012 Information and communications development: Maximizing mobile. 2012; http://siteresources.worldbank.org/EXTINFORMATIONANDCOM MUNICATIONANDTECHNOLOGIES/Resources/IC4D-2012-Report.pdf.

140. Dolan PL. Older patients join crowd consulting Dr. Internet. American Medical News. *American Medical News.* October 22, 2012. http://www.ama-assn.org/amednews/2012/10/22/bisb1022.htm. Accessed February 1, 2013.

141. Singh H, Fox SA, Petersen NJ, Shethia A, Street RL, Jr. Older patients' enthusiasm to use electronic mail to communicate with their physicians: cross-sectional survey. *J Med Internet Res.* 2009;11(2):e18.

142. van den Berg N, Schumann M, Kraft K, Hoffmann W. Telemedicine and telecare for older patients-A systematic review. *Maturitas.* Oct 2012;73(2):94-114.

143. Burke B. *Gamification: Engagement Strategies for Business and IT.* Gartner Inc;November 20, 2012.

144. Christakis NA, Fowler JH. The spread of obesity in a large social network over 32 years. *N Eng J Med.* Jul 26 2007;357(4):370-379.

145. Health Research Institute. *Healthcare unwired: New business models delivering care anywhere.* PriceWaterhouseCoopers;September 2010.

146. GSMA. *Sub-Saharan Africa Mobile Observatory 2012 Report.* 2012.

147. Berry EA. Big insurers investing in mobile health apps. *American Medical News.* January 23, 2012. http://www.amednews.com/article/20120123/business/30123 9959/7/.

148. Dunbrack LA. *Essential Partner Strategies for mHealth.* IDCHealth Insights;September 2012.

149. Broderick A, Lindeman D. *Scaling Telehealth: Lessons from Early Adopters.* The Commonwealth Fund;January 30, 2013.

150. NEHI. *FAST: Detailed Technology Analysis Home Telehealth.* June 2009.

151. PwC Health Resources Institute. Healthcare Unwired. 2010.

152. World Health Organization. *Telemedicine: Opportunities and Developments in Member States.* 2010.

153. Watson T. *2012 Onsite Health Center Survey Report.* 2012.

154. Matt ST. WellPoint expands telemedicine opportunities for doctors. *American Medical News.* January 31, 2013. http://www.amednews.com/article/20130130/business/13013 9999/8/. Accessed January 30, 2013.

155. Courneya PT, Palattao KJ, Gallagher JM. HealthPartners' online clinic for simple conditions delivers savings of $88 per episode and high patient approval. *Health Aff (Millwood).* Feb 2013;32(2):385-392.

156. Integrated Benefits Institute. *Poor Health Costs US Economy $576 Billion.* September 12, 2012.

157. Qualcomm. *Delivering Accountable Care with Remote Monitoring for Chronic Disease Management.* 2012.

158. Bailey JL, BK J. Telementoring: using the Kinect and Microsoft Azure to save lives. *Int J Electronic Finance.* 2013;7:33-47.

159. National Telehealth Policy Resource Center. *State Telehealth Laws and Reimbursement Policies: A Comprehensive Scan of the 50 States and the District of Columbia.* 2013.

160. mHealth Alliance. *Advancing the Dialogue on Mobile Finance and Mobile Health: Country Case Studies.* March 2002.

161. International Telecommunications Union. Statistics. 2011; www.itu.int/ ITU-D/ict/statistics. Accessed February 26, 2013.

162. The United Nations Foundation. mHealth for Development: The Opportunity For Mobile Technology For Health Care In The Developing World. 2009; http://unpan1.un.org/intradoc/groups/public/documents/unpa n/unpan037268.pdf. Accessed March 1, 2013.

163. Koriwchak MJ. Commentary: The economic lessons of mHealth. *mHIMSS.* 2013. http://www.mhimss.org/news/commentary-economic-lessons-mhealth. Accessed March 21, 2013.

164. Labrique AB. Connecting People, Compressing Time and Creating Opportunities: The Promise of Mobile Health. 2012; https://hit.umbc.edu/news/23-connecting-people-compressing-time-and-creating-opportunities-the-promise-of-mobile-health-by-alain-b-labrique. Accessed March 1, 2013.

165. Mahmud N, Rodriguez J, Nesbit J. A text message-based intervention to bridge the healthcare communication gap in the rural developing world. *Technology and health care : official journal of the European Society for Engineering and Medicine.* 2010;18(2):137-144.

166. International Development Research Centre. ICT for health: Empowering Health Workers to Save Lives. 2011; http://www.healthnet.org/uhin. Accessed March 1, 2013.

167. World Health Organization. Maternal Mortality: Fact Sheet 348. May 2012; http://www.who.int/mediacentre/factsheets/fs348/en/index.html. Accessed March 5, 2013.

168. Tamrat T, Kachnowski S. Special delivery: an analysis of mHealth in maternal and newborn health programs and their outcomes around the world. *Matern Child Health J.* Jul 2012;16(5):1092-1101.

169. Book CF. Malawi. 2013; https://www.cia.gov/library/publications/the-world-factbook/geos/mi.html Accessed March 1, 2013.

170. mHealth Alliance. Sustainable Financing for Mobile Health. February 2013; http://www.mhealthalliance.org/images/content/sustainable_fin ancing_for_mhealth_report.pdf. Accessed March 3, 2013.

171. The Telenor Group. mHealth partnership supports mother-infant health. http://www.telenor.com/corporate-responsibility/initiatives-worldwide/mhealth-partnership-supports-motherinfant-health/. Accessed March 8, 2013.

172. Mobile Alliance for Maternal Action. MAMA Overview. 2013; http://healthunbound.org/mama/overview. Accessed February 23, 2013.

173. Chib A. *Information and Communication Technologies for Health Care: Midwife Mobile-Phone Project in Aceh Besar World Vision Endline Report.* 2008.

174. Lund S HM. Wired mothers: Use of mobile phones to improve maternal and neonatal health in Zanzibar. http://www.oresund.org/logistics/content/download/74534/42 9853/file/Ida%20Marie%20Boas_Wired%20Mothers.pdf. Accessed March 8, 2013.

175. Lund S, Hemed M, Nielsen BB, et al. Mobile phones as a health communication tool to improve skilled attendance at delivery in Zanzibar: a cluster-randomised controlled trial. *BJOG.* Sep 2012;119(10):1256-1264.

176. Centers for Disease Control and Prevention. Global Health: Measles, Rubella, CRS. 2012;

http://www.cdc.gov/globalhealth/measles/. Accessed March 9, 2013.

177. World Health Organization. State of the world's vaccines and immunization. Third edition. 2009. 2009; http://www.who.int/immunization/sowvi/en/. Accessed March 9, 2013.

178. Wakadha H, Chandir S, Were EV, et al. The feasibility of using mobile-phone based SMS reminders and conditional cash transfers to improve timely immunization in rural Kenya. *Vaccine.* Jan 30 2013;31(6):987-993.

179. Immunization Rates Rising Using mPhones. *Federal Telecommunizations News.* May 23, 2012. http://telemedicinenews.blogspot.com/2012/05/immunization-rates-rising-using-mphones.html. Accessed June 18, 2013.

180. Positive Innovation for the Next Generation. Disease Surveillance and Mapping. http://www.pingsite.org/tech-projects/disease-surveillance-project/. Accessed March 3, 2013.

181. Drell L. How Mobile Phones Are Saving Lives in the Developing World. *Mashable.* June 8, 2011. http://mashable.com/2011/06/08/sms-medical-startups/. Accessed March 9, 2013.

182. mHIMSS. Health eVillages launches new mHealth initiative in Africa. October 18, 2012; http://www.mhimss.org/news/health-evillages-launches-new-mhealth-initiative-africa. Accessed March 5, 2013.

183. AMREF. AMREF unveils mLearning Project. http://www.amref.org/news/amref-unveils-mlearning-project/?keywords=mhealth. Accessed March 7, 2013.

184. Parham GP, Mwanahamuntu MH, Pfaendler KS, et al. eC3--a modern telecommunications matrix for cervical cancer prevention in Zambia. *J Low Genit Tract Dis.* Jul 2010;14(3):167-173.

185. UNAIDS. Regional fact sheet 2012. 2012; http://www.unaids.org/en/media/unaids/contentassets/documents/epidemiology/2012/gr2012/2012_FS_regional_ssa_en.pdf. Accessed March 2, 1013.

186. World Health Organization. *Towards universal access: scaling up priority HIV/AIDS interventions in the health sector: Progress report 2010.* 2010.

187. Benjamin P. mHealth: Hope or Hype? Experiences from Cell-Life. In: Donner J, Mechael P, eds. *MHealth in Practice: Mobile Technology for Health Promotion in the Developing World*. London: Bloomsbury Academic; 2013.

188. World Health Organization. Strategic Use Of HIV Medicines Could Help End Transmission Of Virus [press release]. http://www.who.int/mediacentre/news/releases/2012/hiv_med ication_20120718/en/index.html. Accessed March 1, 2013.

189. Ivers LC, Kendrick D, Doucette K. Efficacy of antiretroviral therapy programs in resource-poor settings: a meta-analysis of the published literature. *Clinical infectious diseases : an official publication of the Infectious Diseases Society of America*. Jul 15 2005;41(2):217-224.

190. Pop-Eleches C, Thirumurthy H, Habyarimana JP, et al. Mobile phone technologies improve adherence to antiretroviral treatment in a resource-limited setting: a randomized controlled trial of text message reminders. *Aids*. Mar 27 2011;25(6):825-834.

191. Tynan M, Babb S, MacNeil A, Griffin M. State smoke-free laws for worksites, restaurants, and bars--United States, 2000-2010. *MMWR Morbid Mortal Wkly Rep*. Apr 22 2011;60(15):472-475.

192. Haberer JE, Kahane J, Kigozi I, et al. Real-time adherence monitoring for HIV antiretroviral therapy. *AIDS Behav*. Dec 2010;14(6):1340-1346.

193. Angell SY, Cobb LK, Curtis CJ, Konty KJ, Silver LD. Change in trans fatty acid content of fast-food purchases associated with New York City's restaurant regulation: a pre-post study. *Ann Intern Med*. Jul 17 2012;157(2):81-86.

194. Siedner MJ, Lankowski A, Musinga D, et al. Optimizing Network Connectivity for Mobile Health Technologies in sub-Saharan Africa. *PloS One*. 2012;7(9):e45643.

195. Hsiao CJ, Jha AK, King J, Patel V, Furukawa MF, Mostashari F. Office-Based Physicians Are Responding To Incentives And Assistance By Adopting And Using Electronic Health Records. *Health Aff (Millwood)*. Jul 9 2013.

196. Reflexive Practice. Reflexive Practice Web Blog. *Reflexive Practice Web Blog*2013.

197. GSMA mWomen Programme. *Case Study: Vodafone Qatar's Al Johara: Empowerment through Entrepreneurship*.

198. Verbatim Proceedings. Department of Public Health. Connecticut Health Information Technology and Exchange. *Connecticut*

Department of Public Health,. East Hartford, CT: Connecticut Department of Public Health; January 7, 2013.

199. Scott JC. *Domination and the Arts of Resistance : Hidden Transcripts.* First ed. New Haven, CT: Yale University Press; 1992.

200. *mHealth Drivers & Barriers – 2012 Survey: Healthcare Overview.* Medullan;2012.

201. Ask JA. *Building a Pervasive Corporate Mobile Competency.* Forrester;January 25, 2013.

202. The Commonwealth Fund. *Case Studies in Telehealth Adoption.* January 2013.

203. Sharpe R. Many health apps are based on flimsy science at best, and they often do not work. *Washington Post.* November 12, 2012.

204. Ferrero NA, Morrell DS, Burkhart CN. Skin scan: a demonstration of the need for FDA regulation of medical apps on iPhone. *J Am Acad Dermatol.* Mar 2013;68(3):515-516.

205. Stone SP, Fuller C, Savage J, et al. Evaluation of the national Cleanyourhands campaign to reduce Staphylococcus aureus bacteraemia and Clostridium difficile infection in hospitals in England and Wales by improved hand hygiene: four year, prospective, ecological, interrupted time series study. *BMJ (Clinical research ed.).* 2012;344:e3005).

206. Hueussner KM. Mobile health in 2013: From the gym to the doctor's office. *Washington Post* December 26, 2012.

207. Federal Communications Commission. April 3, 2012; http://transition.fcc.gov/Daily_Releases/Daily_Business/2012/db0719/DOC-315316A2.txt. Accessed April 24, 2013.

208. Young S. Are Your Doctor's Hands Clean? This Wristband Knows. *MIT Technology Review.* March 25, 2013.